I0707441

Cannabis (Marijuana) Pharmacy OIL and Cookbook

2 Books in 1

Properties, Strains, Medical Usage, THC and CBD

QUICK and SIMPLE Recipes

BY

DOREEN WEED

© Copyright 2020 Doreen Weed

All rights reserved

CANNABIS PHARMACY OIL

Cannabis Properties, Strains, Medical Usage, Thc And Cbd

By

Doreen Weed

© Copyright 2020 Doreen Weed

All rights reserved.

TABLE OF CONTENTS

INTRODUCTION TO CANNABIS..................................13

MODERN HERBAL MEDICINE 17

CANNABIS HISTORY, PROPERTIES AND PRODUCTS.34

MEDICAL CANNABIS: 55

HOW TO CHOOSE AND USE..............................55

CANNABIS PHENOTYPE AND GENOTYPE...............68

CANNABIS STRAINS 77

DIFFERENCE BETWEEN THC AND CBD STRAINS 82

PRODUCTION OF CANNABIS PHARMACY OIL........109

CANNABIS PHARMACY OILS AND ITS USAGE.........123

USEFULNESS OF CANNABIS OIL FOR THE AGED 142

CANNABIS PHARMACY OIL ON PETS 148

NEGATIVE IMPLICATIONS OF CANNABIS ABUSE ON GENERAL AND ORAL HEALTH................................156

RELATED EFFECTS ON USAGE OF CANNABIS PHARMACY OIL...161

IS ALL CANNABIS OIL THE SAME? 180

ALTERNATIVES TO CANNABIS PHARMACY OIL......192

LAWS AND REGULATIONS ON MEDICINAL CANNABIS AROUND THE WORLD.......................................200

RECOMMENDATIONS 225

CONCLUSION..229

WHAT IS CANNABIS 242

How to recognize marijuana CBD and THC...........244

HISTORY OF CANNABIS 246

Hemp for food 259

Hemp for health & body...........................259

Hemp for Fuel...260

The controversy of classifying: hemp vs cannabis .. 260

Hemp seed oil and hemp extract vs cannabis oil.... 261

HOW CANNABIS BENEFITS WOMEN'S GYNECOLOGICAL HEALTH 262

WHAT IS CANNABIS STRESS? 266

Different kinds of strains 268

THE STEP–UP TECHNIQUE...........................274

Palm Mincer...275

So, How Much CBD Should You Take? 276

TCheck Dosage Checker...........................276

What's the Right Dose of CBD? 276

EXPANDING LAWS...277

Volcano Vaporizer 277

Fruity Pebbly 277

CANNABIS DOSING GUIDE 278

Macro (Or Therapeutic) Dose......................278

Standard Dose 279

HOW TO CALCULATE EDIBLE POTENCY 280

General Dosage Guidelines 281

Regularly talk to a medical care expert..........281

HEMP SEEDS FOR WEIGHT LOSS 283

HEMP HEARTS VS HEMP SEEDS 284

Understand CBD as well as THC Contents....286

Just how exactly hemp seeds support weight loss?...288

Best ways to lose weight with cannabis seeds........293

SOME BENEFITS OF HEMP SEEDS........................295

HOW TO MAKE CSB BROWNIES 299

Non-Vegan CBD brownie 299

Vegan CBD Brownies 301

CBD brownies with vaped buds.........................302

CBD brownies with Cannabis butter.....................302

CANNABIS COCKTAIL SYRUPS............................303

Thai High...303

SIP IT UP...304

Smoke with Spices....................................304

Lime wedge to prepare................................304

WANDERER 305

Marijuana Milk (sugar-free) 305

Vanilla Cannabis Milkshake. 306

STRAWBERRY CANNA-BASIL LEMONADE 307

Marijuana Thai Iced Tea 308

Cup Of Unsweetened Cocoa Powder 308

Hot Canna-Buttered Apple Cider. 309

Sparkling Pear Prosecco Canna Punch 310

Cannabis Olive Oil 311

HOW TO MAKE STONER SWEETS 313

POT CHEF 314

VINAIGRETTE 314

STUFFED STONED JALAPEÑO POPPERS 315

SATIVA SHRIMP SPRING ROLLS WITH MANGO SAUCE.
.... 317

MARIJUANA GUACAMOLE 319

MINI KIND VEGGIE BURRITOS 320

PICO DE GANJA AND NACHOS 322

BRUSCHETTA 323

KIND BUD BRUSCHETTA WITH POT PESTO 324

Marijuana Pancakes 324

MEAT LOAF 325

Cannabis Spinach 326

Marijuana Baked Salmon 327

Marijuana Joe Sandwiches...........................327

Cannabis Balsamic Vinaigrette 328

Sautéed squash 329

Marijuana Spaghetti 329

Marijuana Pepper and Artichoke Dip 330

CANNABIS POTATO AND OLIVE OIL SOUP 331

Cannabis Alfredo Pasta Sauce 331

Marijuana Chili 332

Cannabis Turkey Stuffing 333

Cannabis Caesar Salad 334

Marijuana Crab Stuffed Mushrooms. 335

Marijuana Flour.....................................336

Cannabis Olivia.....................................336

Cannabis Fried Butter Ball..........................337

Marijuana pie N Chicken............................338

Potatoe Mash.......................................339

CANNABIS PIZZA....................................340

Cannabis Salsa N Papaya............................341

Cannabis Salmon 342

Marijuana Salmon Mapple..........................343

Marijuana Tilapia Tacos....................................344

Baked Cannabis Tilapia....................................345

Cannabis Hash Brown Casserole...........................345

Marijuana Baked Pizza Sandwich..........................346

Marijuana BBQ Beef Sandwiches...........................347

Marijuana Basil Chicken Pasta 348

Cannabis Basil Shrimp Pasta 349

Cannabis Tea 350

CANNABIS SHOTS-JELLO....................................352

Marijuana Cupcakes......................................353

Cannabis Brownies.......................................354

BUTTER..356

Cannabis Apple Pecan Galaxy Cake.......................357

Cannabis Chocolate Pudding 357

Cannabis Cashew Cookies 358

Cannabis Sugar Cookie 359

Velvet Cupcakes...360

Marijuana Oatmeal Cookies. 361

Canna Lemon Bread......................................361

Orange Cake 362

Chocolate Milkshake 363

Banana Blueberry Healthy Smoothie 363

Cinnamon Coffee Cake 364

Canna Flat Bread 365

Tiramisu Milk Shake....................................366

Cannabis Bread 367

Canna Extra Pound Cake..............................367

Marijuana scones 368

Sugar Squares...369

Delicious Chocolate Space Cake 370

Marijuana Cheesecake.................................371

Marijuana Truffles 372

Chocolate Chip Cookies 373

Cannabis Pumpkin Muffins 374

Marijuana Orange Dark Chocolate Chip Cookies.....375

Marijuana Cranberry and also Macadamia Nut Cookies
....376

Health Bars...377

Marijuana Caramel Walnut Dream Bars 378

Iced Marshmallow Cookies 378

Marijuana Brown-eyes..................................379

Marijuana Peanut Butter Cup Cookies...................380

Marijuana Butterscotch Space Pops.....................381

CONCLUSION 383

INTRODUCTION TO CANNABIS

Cannabis is a plant that is a noteworthy wellspring of confusion for a few. While realities show that a couple of kinds of hemp are unlawful as a result of the substance THC, which is a psychoactive molecule, not the total of the sorts of Hemp contain THC. Cannabis oil got prominence with the prosperity mindful of the world during the 1990s. For an impressive period of time people used oil until it was removed from the market since oil is delivered utilizing the seeds of the cannabis plant. The DEA endeavored to express that the oil was illegal, anyway in HIA versus DEA it was settled that hemp based sustenance things, including Cannabis oil were cleared from the Controlled Substances Act.

Today, Cannabis oil returns to a seat at the most noteworthy purpose of the universe of sustenance and the remedial world. It is basic to observe that there are a couple of different sorts of Cannabis oil. There is an expeller pressed grouping, which is a sustenance type thing. It is used in sustenance and embellishing specialists. Likewise, steam distilled major oil is made using the hemp seed, which is also used in the area of excellence in care and fragrance based treatment practices. This is the expeller pressed sustenance thing we are talking about. The use of the Marijuana plant started in China about 2300 B.C.

According to Chinese time-thought, the plant contains the solution for endlessness. The Chinese similarly used Cannabis oil to treat Malaria, menstrual issues and productivity. In the 10th century, Indians began to use the oil to treat indigestion, and anorexia similarly to external wounds and infections, asthma, menstrual torment and anything is possible from that point. The plant fiber was used to produce textiles, sails and ropes until the start of this century. Nonetheless, taking into account the genuine concern that it is usually pleasing, various interactions will eventually make the hemp strands surface.

Cannabis oil is rich with unsaturated fats and fundamental unsaturated fats. Around 30-35% of the greatness of the hemp seeds is the oil, which is crushed out in the age of the oil. The oil contains the essential unsaturated fats OMEGA-3 and OMEGA-6 at a perfect high rate, many equivalents to chest milk. The oil in like manner contains protein, central supplements and minerals, which makes it an ideal dietary improvement. Fundamental unsaturated fats are the establishments of authentic sustenance rebuilding and repairing the body from infection. To be sure, even in the excellence care items industry, Cannabis oil drives the way. Clinical studies have shown that Cannabis oil is particularly amazing in recovering extraordinary skin issue, for instance, atopic dermatitis quite far up to devours.

Hemp oil sustains the protected structure, keeps up a strong cardiovascular system, and is amazing in helping the body fight a not unimportant once-over of conditions, for instance, cutting down *horrendous* cholesterol, raising *incredible* cholesterol, cutting down heartbeat and decreasing the threat of respiratory disappointment, similarly as being quieting. In case you are a danger sufferer and are encountering chemotherapy, using Cannabis oil is recommended all the while. It invigorates sound cell creation and decreases the damage to the body on account of treatment. The oil doesn't battle with ordinary restorative drugs and is not a fix, yet rather is complimentary. In 1995, Deborah Gez made Moriah Herbs, and brought more than thirty years of experience to the field of home developed drug. Moriah Herbs is a pioneer in aroma based treatment, central oils and home developed repairing.

MODERN HERBAL MEDICINE

The use of plants as medicines originates from human history and archeological evidence shows that during the Paleolithic (around sixty thousand years before) we used restorative plants. In Mesopotamia the Sumerians made mud tablets with arrangements of many restorative plants, (for example, myrrh and opium) and the Ancient Egyptians composed the Ebers Papyrus around 1500 BC, which contains data on more than eight-hundred-fifty plant medicines, including garlic, juniper, cannabis, castor bean, aloe, and mandrake. In India the utilization of herbs to treat infirmities shapes an enormous piece of Ayurvedic prescription and obviously everybody knows about how plants and herbs are utilized widely in conventional Chinese Medicine.

The Greeks brought herbalism into the cutting edge age and evacuated a significant part of the supernatural quality and enchantment which were available in prior writings. Hippocrates specifies two-hundred-fifty helpful herbs in his incredible works, and a Greek Physician named Dioscorides distributed a book called De Materia

Medica which contained more than six-hundred restorative plants. Another Greek Galen delivered itemized abstracts on medication which included in excess of six-hundred plants and these were deciphered and counseled by doctors the world over for a long time. All through the Medieval time frame physical and otherworldly wellbeing kept on being upheld for the most part with plants and herbs. This treatment was typically done by priests and nuns who gave nursing administrations, with the Benedictine religious communities known for their top to bottom learning of herbals. They tended nurseries that developed the herbs which were viewed as helpful for the treatment of the different human ills. The priests additionally invested a lot of their energy deciphering old style chips away at herbalism into Latin and creating *Herbals* to be utilized by doctors.

The fifteenth, sixteenth, and seventeenth hundreds of years were the extraordinary period of herbals, huge numbers of them accessible without precedent for English and different dialects instead of Latin or Greek. Close by the customary acts of Herbalism there were many learned men of science and prescription who accepted sickness was brought about by *terrible humor* in the body that must be driven out and discharged. The popular American specialist Benjamin Rush, Treasurer of the Mint, and endorser of the Declaration of Independence, wrote numerous restorative course books, in which he prescribed splashing patients with cold water in the winter, spinning patients from ropes suspended from the roof for a considerable length of time, just as beating, starving and obnoxiously mishandling patients. He additionally poured corrosive on their backs and cut them with blades enabling the injuries to be kept open for a considerable length of time or years, to encourage *"perpetual release of awful humor from the cerebrum"*.

When King Charles II woke up feeling sick his Royal Barber took sixteen ounces of blood, and his primary care physicians depleted a further eight ounces. He was made to swallow antimony, a poisonous metal, and given a progression of bowel purges. At the point when his sickness proceeded with Charles' head was shaved and rankling operators were applied to his scalp, to drive the awful humor descending. Pigeon droppings were applied to the bottoms of Charles' feet, and more blood was drawn. He was given white sugar treats, to float his spirits, and nudged with a super hot poker. He was then given fourty drops of seepage from *"the skull of a man that was rarely covered"* what it's identity was, guaranteed, had kicked the bucket a roughest passing. At long last, squashed stones from the inner parts of a goat from East India were constrained down his throat. Charles II kicked the bucket on 1685 February 6th.

In the eighteenth century anyway doctors tried to turn out to be progressively logical and there were numerous self-prepared stylist specialists, pharmacists, maternity specialists, medicate vendors, and pretenders who were rehearsing medicine right now. In any case, the town Wise Women could in any case be depended on to supply customary herbs or blends to treat minor sicknesses and this training kept on being prevalent with the common laborers who couldn't bear to pay doctor's expenses. Samuel Thomson was a self-instructed ranch kid who took in herbalism from a nearby shrewd lady and composed a book enumerating these techniques, this book was well known to the point that pretty much every home had a duplicate (together with a book of scriptures) and it was even taken on wagon-prepares and conveyed over the USA.

The American Medical Association came into control towards the finish of the nineteenth Century and the logical insurgency lessened the prevalence of herbalism and presented a time of perilous medical practices presented by the recently framed pharmaceutical industry. During this period Paracelsus presented the utilization of dynamic synthetic medications (like arsenic, copper sulfate, iron, mercury, and sulfur). On the off chance that you were a focus on nineteenth century mother you could now buy for your kids a progression of *alleviating syrups*, tablets and powders which in reality contained hazardous opiates, for example, morphine sulfate, chloroform, morphine hydrochloride, codeine, heroin, powdered opium, and cannabis indica," and some of the time a few of them in mix. Heroin was likewise usually used to treat hacks.

Mercury was utilized much of the time to treat numerous normal infirmities. Mercury, as we presently know, is dangerous to the body and side effects of mercury harming incorporate chest agonies, heart and lung issues, hacking, tremors, savage muscle fits, insane responses, incoherence, pipedreams, and even self-destructive inclinations! Numerous post-mortem examinations uncovered *Silver Liver Syndrome* to be the reason for death during this period. Present day medicine then *advanced* considerably more to incorporate radical medications like phlebotomy, leeches, and exploratory techniques like lobotomies and electric stun medicines. Trepanation, boring openings in the head, was another well known treatment and was most ordinarily utilized for seizures and headaches!

Diet pills were presented during the 1920s and '30s which were in truth containers loaded up with got dried out tapeworms or tapeworm eggs. In the 1950s and 1960s new pills were being sold that vowed to soften away those pounds and inches yet these could cause fevers, heart inconveniences, visual deficiency, demise and birth abandons. Those eating routine pills were massively addictive and in truth contained unadulterated amphetamines. Since the beginning of current medicine, the pharmaceutical business has fortunately advanced and controls are set up to guarantee pharmaceutical medications and medicines are ok for us to utilize. Without a doubt physician recommended medications can spare and change lives. I entirely support and embrace that you keep on utilizing any professionally prescribed medicine which you might be at present taking and ought not to quit ingesting any recommended medications without counseling your primary care physician first.

In any case, it is irrefutable that close by the advantages which physicians recommended medications can offer they can likewise accompany unwelcome symptoms. Record quantities of patients are enduring or kicking the bucket because of physician endorsed medication symptoms. Some generally recorded and demonstrated symptoms from physician recommended medications extend from cerebral pains, tiredness, skin responses, stoppage, looseness of the bowels, gastrointestinal issues, stomach hurts, water gauge addition, joint and muscle torment and diminished authority over real works, loss of taste, amnesia, locate misfortune, mental trips, sickness and heaving causing lack of hydration, inner draining and oesophageal break, through to unfavorably susceptible responses that can deliver an anaphylactic reaction in patients, serious torment, aggregate or incomplete loss of motion, strokes, muscle agony and loss of muscle co-appointment, blood clusters, coronary episodes, congestive cardiovascular breakdown, deep rooted heart harm and cardiomyopathy and incredibly even malignant growth. Physician endorsed medications have additionally been connected to misery and self-destructive contemplations.

Well that is a significant not insignificant rundown of realized reactions from taking physician endorsed medications, and this is in no way, shape or form a total list! You will locate a comparable rundown of perilous known symptoms from the synthetic substances found in our regular family unit items - the normal American home contains more than 63 dangerous items including antiperspirants and antiperspirants, scents, toilet bowl cleaners, over-the-counter meds, pills, creams, gels and so on., healthy skin items, and *deodorizers*. These items contain many synthetic mixes that are conceivably perilous.

Numerous ordinary items like cleansers and shampoos, cleaning up fluid or air pocket shower, even toothpaste, in certainty anything which froths, as often as possible contains a fixing known as Sodium Lauryl Ether Sulfate which can cause extreme skin and eye aggravation, loose bowels, sensory system melancholy, worked breathing and in uncommon cases demise. Parabens are another basic fixing we can discover in shampoos, business creams, shaving gels, individual ointments, topical/parenteral pharmaceuticals, shower tanning arrangement, cosmetics, and toothpaste and are likewise typical nourishment added substance. Parabens have been appeared to cause skin bothering and contact dermatitis and rosacea in people with paraben hypersensitivities and all the more worryingly they can impersonate the female hormone estrogen and have been found in bosom malignancy tumors and connected with the early beginning of pubescence in young ladies.

Another lethal fixing found in numerous family unit cleaners is Butoxyethanol which whenever assimilated through the skin can harm your blood, liver and kidneys and another concoction which is known to cause kidney harm is Perchloroethylene which is usually found in cover cleaners. A fixing found in window cleaning arrangements is Diethylene Glycol is known to discourage the sensory system and most toilet cleaners contain a large group of unsafe synthetic compounds and acids which could cause visual impairment in a flash, and are harmful to the respiratory and circulatory frameworks. Maybe one of the most stunning contaminations in our house is the regularly utilized deodorizers which contain substances called phthalates (articulated Thalates), which are incredibly perilous and known to cause hormonal variations from the norm, conceptive issues and even birth absconds. Worryingly the names on all these regular ordinary family items are frequently deceptive and mistaking for bundling proposing items are *all common*, and so forth when in truth they contain various poisons.

Obviously, there is presently a developing pattern to utilize increasingly normal items in our homes and on our bodies. Numerous individuals are deliberately detoxing their homes and ways of life by coming back to customary strategies and by and by making our own cleaning items, excellence items, and individual care items like toothpaste, cleanser, face cream just as utilizing unadulterated normal items like plants and herbs by and by to battle minor illnesses and advance great health.

Presently, in these modern occasions it would be hard for us to turn the clock back as we may wish and recapture the learning once went from age to age about how to utilize Mother Nature's plants and herbs to keep up our great health and stay away from the requirement for conceivably lethal synthetic concoctions in our ordinary family unit and excellence items and physician recommended drugs. Quite a bit of that information has been lost and a significant number of those fixings and strategies would not be useful for us to utilize any more.

So, What Decisions Do We Have On The Off Chance That We Need To Bring Our Families Up In An Increasingly Common Manner?

Numerous individuals have found humankind's most productive technique for rehearsing herbalism - they utilize 100% unadulterated basic oils, which contain the *soul of the plants*. Basic oils are the exceptionally focused, fragrant embodiments of trees, bushes, herbs, grasses, gums and blooms. Restorative evaluation oils can be utilized fragrantly either legitimately breathed in or diffused, topically (applied to the skin), or now and again taken inside (ingested). The oils all have their own novel dynamic properties and by and large, every basic oil contains more than hundred constituents with all the more being found each day. one drop of unadulterated fundamental oil contains fourty million trillion particles that influence the body at the cell level. Every day, an ever-increasing number of people are changing to a cleaner way of life with fewer poisons in their homes and, like our precursors, we are actually adapting how to use the restorative properties of herbs and plants. We make our own cleaning items utilizing economical basic fixings in mix with basic oils, we make our very own self consideration items, for example, cleansers, shower salts, toothpaste, mouthwash, cleanser, child wipes, creams, and in reality each item you presently use can be imitated in a protected, common structure utilizing fundamental oils related to items like Epsom salts, olive oil, coconut oil, dark colored sugar, ocean salt, vinegar, refined water, and so on.

Right now there is an oily upset occurring, each day an ever increasing number of homes choose to come back to progressively customary attempted and tried strategies for homemaking and health the board. With the monstrous development that fundamental oils are encountering as we come back to utilizing more straightforward and progressively normal items in our home, there has been an ascent in modest *off the rack* impersonation basic oils which are not Therapeutic Grade oils, and are just appropriate to be utilized for their scent. A fundamental oil can legitimately be marked "unadulterated" regardless of whether it contains as meager as 5% of the genuine oil (that is just 5% of the dynamic elements of the oil). The rest of the jug is regularly loaded up with modest engineered filler synthetic compounds which have been delivered for their *scent* characteristics as it were. These oils regularly contain hurtful synthetic concoctions and potential poisons. Stay away from items named *scent* or *parfum* as these are second rate aroma grade basic oils and may contain possibly hurtful sulfates or phthalates.

Basic Oils make them flabbergast properties which advance great health and bolster the body's common protections, they bolster the safe framework, are state of mind hoisting, fragrant, unwinding, renewing, oxygenating, purging, they help cell recovery, are high in cancer prevention agents, support stamina and vitality, improve mental lucidity, help oversee uneasiness and dissatisfaction, and advance generally speaking prosperity, essentialness, and life span!

So to summarize humankind has been using the intensity of Mother Nature's plants and herbs to advance great health and prosperity for more than sixty thousand years. In the last barely any hundred years this information has gotten to some degree lost to numerous individuals as we have experienced a time of logical revelations, and medical leaps forward and these customary home grew plans and techniques have gotten to some degree outdated. Nonetheless, there is a renaissance occurring and consistently an ever increasing number of individuals are searching out an elective decision. The prevalence of conventional home grew plans and healthy home-made cures are developing each day. Fundamental oils are the most productive, compelling and minimal effort way that enables us to pick a progressively regular and customary way of life for our families. There is an oily transformation occurring right now as we each try to get back in agreement with Mother Nature.

Misguided judgments About Alternative Medicine

Medical marijuana or MMJ has been utilized throughout recent decades to help individuals beset with genuine medical conditions that incorporate, yet are not restricted to glaucoma, malignancy, epilepsy, AIDS, and MS (Multiple Sclerosis). As one of the best specialists that assist individuals with adapting to incessant agony, medical marijuana offers patients help from extraordinary distress by easing their side effects. Understanding the science behind the adequacy of marijuana is significant so as to scatter these fantasies and settle on a very much educated decision about what it really offers. When managed under the supervision of a certified and able specialist or medical expert, medical marijuana lessens the torment and queasiness that different health issues cause. Scores of individuals accept that medical marijuana is very addictive and it builds the reliance on the medication.

Research shows that there is no proof to help this conviction in light of the fact that to begin with, medical cannabis does not have any synthetic concoctions that may trigger habit in individuals who use it as a piece of their treatment procedure. At that point there are different confusions that MMJ may likewise prompt the utilization of hard drugs, for example, cocaine and like the previous, this is additionally only a misinterpretation. While medical marijuana can be smoked, this isn't the main way that it tends to be utilized. Directly from doctor prescribed drugs and pills that contain manufactured types of medical marijuana to other substitute treatment strategies, cannabinoids, for example, THC can be conveyed to the body without smoking MMJ. The blooms and leaves can be absorbed a blend of liquor to remove the cannabinoids in marijuana. This mixture can either be added to beverages and nourishment or consumed through skin patches and in this structure; it takes MMJ as meager as a half hour to create the ideal impact. The dynamic parts can likewise be moved into cooking oil and spread by stewing the plant in them for a few hours. This is typically used to heat treats and brownies or make different sorts of nourishment that a patient may discover tantalizing.

Thought there are tests that show that Medical cannabis can cause momentary memory misfortune in certain patients who are experiencing treatment, actually the impact is just impermanent. Medical marijuana neither decreases their knowledge nor does it influence their long haul memory. Despite the fact that medical cannabis is an all-common substance that is gotten from plants, the misguided judgments about it are very dubious and ridiculous.

CANNABIS HISTORY, PROPERTIES AND PRODUCTS

For many years, cannabis has been associated with humanity. Cannabis has characteristics that are psychoactive and remedial. In nature, the cannabis plant can grow up to five meters in height. It blooms in late harvest time between the fag end of the mid-year season. Some of the Chinese records written in 2800 BC were the most reliable reference to cannabis. In many Asian nations, cannabis is a wild plant. Cannabis is broadly esteemed to have begun in India. Numerous indigenous networks over the world have been utilizing cannabis for a few purposes like strict, recreational, and medical. Numerous doctors recommend meds having cannabis to patients experiencing such sicknesses as glaucoma, different sclerosis, HIV, and malignant growth, other than a few others. Cannabis in like manner gives the vim to the heart and the results have been exhibited to be a lot of equivalent to an individual rehearsing reliably in the diversion focus.

Nowadays, cannabis is perceived as a drug. Cannabis is precluded in various countries. Normally, cannabis customers prevented from securing the medicine have been viewed as commanding in nature. Toward the day's end, cannabis is addictive rationally. The effect is extremely similar to steroids that are anabolic in nature. What is more, addicts of a couple of hard medications have been viewed as the wellsprings of major sociological or health issues. However, an assessment has exhibited that cannabis customers are less disposed to make such aggravations. More than 400 manufactured mixes set up cannabis. Cannabis has been used by various indigenous people because of its psychoactive effects. The fundamental psychoactive segment in cannabis is 'THC' or tetrahydrocannabinol.

A lot of cannabis brown haze can antagonistically influence the circulatory strain process and an individual can even black out because of this impact. Individuals having a history of such health issues like dissemination and heart issue, other than schizophrenia should absolutely evade cannabis. Such individuals can have inconveniences regardless of whether they become uninvolved smokers. Routine cannabis smokers experience the evil impacts of lung threat, emphysema, and bronchitis. Thusly, the best way to deal with go without being a cannabis aficionado is to express 'NO!' to the medicine the main go through ever. There is reliably the threat of a standard cannabis customer taking to progressively destructive psychoactive medications like cocaine and heroin.

The cannabis plant is commonly referred to as hemp, marijuana or cannabis indica. Cannabis is called cannabis, tobacco, opium, pot, herb, smoke, vapor, hemp, marijuana, or ganja, unlike the different names.

Many young people around the globe have been seen stuck in marijuana, regardless of the prohibitions.

As cancer-causing agents (specialists that induce malignant growth), marijuana has more tar than tobacco.

The most grounded and focused type of cannabis oil is fabricated from the cannabis sap. The sap is broken down, separated lastly vanished. In the UK, this oil is separated by cocaine and heroin closely and is a prescription under the course of action of Class A. As squares, cannabis tar is removed from the buds of cannabis. When they are prepared for use, these cannabis squares are then warmed up and disintegrated. The shade of the cannabis sap can fluctuate from green to dim dark colored. This structure is prominently called *hash, soapbar* or *dark*. The home grown type of cannabis is known as skunk, weed or just 'grass'. It is set up from the dried or powdered buds of the cannabis plant.

Researches on cannabis have hurled fascinating information. Take for example the discovering around 46% of individuals in the age bunch from fourteen to thirty have been snared to cannabis regardless of whether incidentally. Moreover, 50% of these people have come back to the plant. At this point web surfing in the United States, marijuana smoking was seen as increasingly common. While in the UK, marijuana has been found to have as much as 78% of people kept for medicine-related offenses.

Cannabis is presently the most broadly utilized and dubious medication on the planet. While a few people shout out for stricter marijuana laws and stiffer punishments for clients and sellers, others censure lawful frameworks which rebuff peaceful *pot smokers*. United States residents everything being equal and social statuses expend it, yet American government officials looking for re-appointment are hesitant to advocate its legitimateness. Generally speaking, a superior comprehension of the history, uses, and risks of marijuana can assist social orders with creating progressively productive and vote based arrangements for its guidelines.

In the same way as other personality modifying drugs, marijuana has been utilized worldwide for a large number of years. Antiquated Chinese writings portray its utilization in both recreational and medical settings. Archeological proof proposes that the cannabis plant previously spread from Asia to Africa, and was considered developing to be Europe as right on time as the 6th century, A.D. Over a thousand years after the fact, pilgrim Americans developed hemp as a money crop for its handiness in materials.

Somewhere in the range of 1850 and 1942, American specialists routinely endorsed marijuana for help with discomfort, stomach issues, and joint pain. Cannabis was likewise utilized recreationally - and legitimately - during the majority of this time. It was not until 1935 and the death of the Uniform State Narcotic Drug Act that most states started to carefully direct the medication.

All through the 1950s and 60s, marijuana was seen fundamentally as an insubordinate, countercultural, or ra*dical tranquilize*. However, despite everything it didn't convey the taboos or hardened legitimate punishments that exist today. The 1970 Controlled Substances Act added to the present the norm by making marijuana a Schedule I medicate - in a similar class as heroin, cocaine, and different opiates. As a feature of the Reagan organization's War on Drugs, obligatory condemning laws went during the 1980s which still require sentences of a quarter century or more for thrice-indicted marijuana guilty parties.

These authoritative choices stay questionable right up 'til the present time, and change supporters contend that marijuana isn't about so risky or propensity framing as to require such severe legitimate punishments. They additionally much of the time push for the decriminalization of marijuana, particularly for medical use. Gatherings of these promoters are enormous and assorted, and incorporate such associations as the Coalition for Rescheduling Cannabis, Law Enforcement Against Prohibition, and Students for Sensible Drug Policy.

Notwithstanding varying suppositions on the legitimateness and social agreeableness of marijuana, the vast majority can concur that the quantity of individuals captured for peaceful marijuana wrongdoings has become a significant issue. US correctional facilities are loaded up with a huge number of these convicts, and Congress burns through billions of citizen dollars keeping them bolted up. Besides, these guilty parties are regularly put in indistinguishable offices from killers, vicious street pharmacists, and different risky lawbreakers. They face long, life-expending sentences, and even marijuana clients who need assistance with dependence seldom approach appropriate treatment programs. Increasingly more marijuana clients wind up in the slammer, however the medication issue in America isn't improving.

Fortunately, help is accessible for the individuals who need it. On the off chance that you are battling with marijuana or other addictive substances, utilize the connections underneath for a classified conference. We are remaining by day and night to kick you off making a course for recuperation.

Properties

Marijuana contains the substance THC which is known by most of individuals yet expected without a compound hint, to be dangerous or addictive. THC, short for some long geeky name you'll easily forget at any rate, has been managed in different sub-atomic structures to malignancy, HIV and various sclerosis sufferers for a considerable length of time with apparent achievement.

Tetrahydrocannabinol (THC) is the dynamic substance in cannabis and is one of the most established psychedelic drugs known. There is proof that cannabis concentrates were utilized by the Chinese as a natural cure since the main century AD. Cannabis originates from the blooming tops and leaves of the hemp plant, Cannabis sativa (appeared in the image on the right). For a considerable length of time this plant has been generally developed far and wide for its filaments, and in reality, the word canvas, which is a material produced using woven hemp strands, takes its name from cannabis. Be that as it may, cannabis is all the more usually known as the wellspring of the marijuana tranquilizes, despite the fact that the word marijuana applies both to the entire plant, and to the sap from it (in spite of the fact that this is now and then likewise called hashish).

Cannabis contains around sixty diverse psychoactive synthetic concoctions called cannabinoids, of which the most significant one is tetrahydrocannabinol (THC). The method of activity of THC is as yet not appropriately comprehended, despite the fact that it is realized that of the two stereoisomers (identical representations), the (-

)- structure (the left-gave type of the particle) is ten-fifteen times more intense than the (+)- structure.

The cannabinoids have a place with a class of synthetic substances called terpenoids, which means terpene-like. These mixes happen as fundamental oils inside numerous plants and some are associated with the development of nutrients, steroids, colors and scents. The fragrance business depends on mixes, for example, these, and they additionally discover an assortment of employments in the nourishment and pharmaceutical industry as flavor and scent improvers. Terpenes can be direct, (for example, geraniol or citronella) or cyclic as in THC. Instances of some other straightforward cyclic terpenes are demonstrated as follows.

Cannabis Products

As cannabis turns out to be increasingly lawful, the industry encompassing it keeps on growing. Government officials presently crusade on a foundation of all out weed authorization since it is that famous a position, and it appears to be each other week there's a neighborhood news anecdote about a mother who turned into a mogul preparing and selling edibles. Since it has arrived at suburbia, organizations need to extend advertising endeavors.

That is in reality entirely troublesome. Noticeable web indexes like Google aren't especially enthused about letting individuals promoting marijuana products on their site, regardless of whether the express it is created in is lawful. Makers have been compelled to discover different intends to sell their products.

Regardless of these barricades, the blast in cannabis fame has implied a blast in cannabis products this decade. Since THC and CBD can enter the body from numerous points of view (smoking, vaping, ingesting, through skin) the quantity of products that can be made with it are, if not perpetual, absolutely abundant. Certain products, however, appear to be progressively noticeable, or possibly on the ascent, then others.

It ought to be noticed that this e-book is not a support of any of the products that will be referenced. Cannabis is as yet illicit at the government level, and because of its characterization as a Schedule 1 medication the measure of research that can be led on it is constrained. This is basically an affirmation of prevalent kinds of products in states where cannabis is lawful in some structure:

1. Cannabis Oil

This is truly a really wide classification in its own right. There are weed products we will get the opportunity to further down that contain cannabidiol (CBD) oil to give you the ideal impacts. Be that as it may, cannabis oil can be taken without anyone else in various structures. That flexibility has made it effectively the most looked for after cannabis product for individuals searching for lawful use. CBD oils have exceedingly low hints of THC, so they won't give you the high that you would typically partner with marijuana. That way one can possibly get the ideal impacts, help with discomfort, uneasiness alleviation, sickness help, and so forth, without psychoactive responses.

Epilepsy is the condition that appears to get the most steady help for utilization of cannabis oil, even governmentally; the U.S. Nourishment and Drug Administration (FDA) as of late got a consistent vote by their government warning council to suggest endorsement of a pharmaceutical CBD oil known as Epidiolex, which can be utilized to treat certain uncommon types of epilepsy. Be that as it may, CBD oil has additionally demonstrated itself to be helpful with respect to relief from discomfort, malignant growth treatment, nervousness, misery, and rest issues, among different conditions.

CBD oil, as its own usable element, can come in a few structures, and the bigger organizations that produce and sell them will offer an assortment of choices to browse. E-fluid for a vape pen is the most widely recognized structure, yet another is tinctures. CBD tinctures are drops of concentrated CBD extricate that are dropped under your tongue and assimilate in the mouth. There are cases as well, which can be taken with water like your normal pill.

Obviously, on the off chance that somebody who needs legitimate cannabis oil likewise does not need a broker, they are allowed to truly simply put CBD oil on their tongue and swallow it. CBD hemp oil is legitimately sold at certain dispensaries.

2. Cannabis Beauty and Skin Care Products

As CBD utilize turned out to be increasingly across the board and cannabis turned out to be additionally sanctioned in more expresses, certain organizations and business visionaries had thoughts of showcasing these products to individuals who aren't regularly promoted weed: rural ladies. Because of this, the industry of CBD beauty products develops exponentially consistently, however it is not simply rural ladies who use them. CBD, notwithstanding the advantages referenced before, is additionally said to have mitigating properties due to cannabinoid receptors in skin. A few researchers state it might have the option to help battle skin break out, and beauty/skincare products with cannabinoids are publicized as having the option to help with relief from discomfort, hydration, or even only an euphoric loosened up feeling.

How standard are these products turning out to be? Products containing CBD are currently being sold on

Sephora's site. The blend of impacts these products indicate to offer are horrendously enticing, all things considered. Cannabis demulcents ointments offer the capability of muscle relief from discomfort, while moisturizers and rubs offer the charm of more clear skin. Shower bombs and shower salts may bring some truly necessary help and unwinding in the tub. The weed topicals market is genuine, and continually extending; you would now be able to purchase marijuana body wash, lip gleam, and mascara as well. The sort of cannabinoids your beauty products have help decide the impacts. A large number of these products center around CBD and the health benefits it gives. Be that as it may, some additionally have more THC, accessible in dispensaries.

3. Cannabis Beverages

Cannabis beverages have not arrived at the standard statures of the beauty products, yet they're getting more presentation, as prove by an ongoing article about CBD mixed drinks in Goop. Mixed drinks implanted with cannabis are still in their early stages, consigned for the most part to a couple of bars in Los Angeles, however should recreational marijuana use keep on getting sanctioned in more expresses, it is a pattern that could grow rapidly. Beverages implanted with marijuana have been consigned to states where the medication is either completely legitimized or decriminalized, acting nearly as test markets for future states. In Colorado, where recreational marijuana is legitimate, a few dispensaries, like Medicine Man, which has various areas - sell cannabis cola and fruit juice. What is more, numerous coffeehouses in New York sell cannabis-implanted espressos, for quieting down any individual who gets a bad case of nerves from a solid cup.

In any case, the one beverage that is regularly given CBD tests, it is lager. This is on the grounds that notwithstanding all the previously mentioned impacts of cannabinoids, the terpenes in cannabis offer various smells and tastes. There have been a few detours en route, especially because of government decisions around what is and is not a Schedule one medication. There have been workarounds however, particularly for brewers and bottling works that stay in states with lawful weed. Keith Villa, maker of Blue Moon, is dealing with cannabis-injected non-fermented lagers in Colorado, while distilleries like Coalition Brewing have CBD lager accessible at select areas in both Oregon and Washington.

4. Cannabis Chocolates

Edibles are an especially well known approach to get high, as they have more strength than different techniques. It likewise allows you to nibble while taking your now legitimate medicine, which is an or more. The most notable edibles are genuinely standard - the weed brownie, the pot treat, marijuana gummies (which have once in a while raised organizations to run into lawful ruckus because of concerns children may unintentionally take them).

As it gets lawful and organizations need to showcase cannabis treats, however, it is chocolates that have become something of a pattern. Chocolates can be showcased to those keen on attempting lawful weed yet who need an increasingly *refined* technique than smoking a joint. It additionally enables organizations to endeavor a more advanced advertising effort than you could do with, say, a sticky bear. Two of the more noticeable producers of marijuana chocolates, Kiva and Défoncé, each utilization a Godiva-esque plan to their wrappers. Presently you can feel extravagant eating a chocolate bar intended to get you high.

These chocolates are sold in restricted style, typically, as they contain THC. Défoncé is just sold and conveyed in California. In any case, should these advertising endeavors stay fruitful, if legitimate marijuana spreads to extra states it won't just be CA dispensaries that stocks them.

5. Cannabis Gummies

Need desserts however not chocolate? Not to stress. Gummies, especially CBD-explicit gummies, have gotten one of the most prevalent products in the wake of legitimate marijuana. In spite of the fact that still in an unregulated area, which means it is difficult to decide with any genuine precision the amount CBD is truly in them, CBD gummies are presently productive enough that it's normal to see CBD sticky worms at a neighborhood service station.

Subsequently, on the off chance that you live in a state with medical marijuana and have a medical marijuana card (or live in a state with lawful recreational marijuana and are of lawful age), your nearby dispensary is sure to have sticky bears, worms and more to look over, regardless of whether with just CBD or with THC too. Organizations like Green Roads and Diamond CBD offer a gathering of CBD gummies for those where weed is lawful. Gummies are effectively one of the most pervasive choices accessible to those searching for a treat.

6. Cannabis Capsules

Not as sweet as the chocolates and gummies or as reviving as a lager, capsules are a possibility for the individuals who simply need something to take care of business. Capsules are increasingly famous for the individuals who aren't searching for a nibble with their weed, deciding to rather take it like medicine, which, to numerous individuals in this nation, is the thing that it is.

Capsules are frequently most mainstream for CBD use. The previously mentioned Medicine Man in Colorado, for instance, sells both CBD capsules and cannabinol (CBN) capsules. Resembling some other case pills, it's as straightforward as anyone might imagine.

7. Cannabis Dog Treats

Is it possible offering cannabis to your pets? Is that sheltered? Well don't give your dog a pot treat with human partitions, and be careful about anything with high THC content, however there are a few organizations that have played with making hemp and CBD products explicitly for pets. Numerous accounts of pets being effectively treated by marijuana are recounted, as getting endorsement for government research into the subject has demonstrated exceedingly troublesome and vets are not lawfully permitted to recommend it. In any case, numerous researchers stay resolved to consider the impacts medical marijuana can have on pets, and some nearby legislators in states like California have acquainted bills with attempt and authorize endorsing cannabis for them.

More inside and out examinations would enable us to decide exactly how evident a significant number of the cases - that CBD can help pet proprietors treat malignant growth, epilepsy, osteoporosis, joint agony, and uneasiness, really are. All things considered, hemp and cannabidiol have not demonstrated themselves to have any exceptional hazard to dogs, as long as you stay mindful; only one out of every odd organization that claims their CBD products have negligible THC is coming clean. An excessive amount of THC isn't useful for dogs. Should you have just chosen to attempt CBD for your puppy's infirmity, there are choices. Canna-pet offer hemp dog treats in a few flavors just as tinctures, which are another prevalent technique for pets as some can be exacting about treats and capsules. Dispensaries in Colorado may likewise sell treats for your dog.

Be that as it may, as referenced, be progressively cautious about cannabis products for your dog. The absence of government guideline or sufficient investigations implies there is no genuine solid assurance of what amount is a lot for dogs. Cannabis products made for pets are made carefully for down to earth purposes; don't get them high.

MEDICAL CANNABIS:
HOW TO CHOOSE AND USE

From little data to an over-burden of data on the web, it is anything but difficult to envision that a great many people living with torment, their relatives, and parental figures will be overpowered about whether cannabis is a reasonable help with discomfort alternative. Most importantly, it is critical to have a genuine discourse and settle on an educated choice, in organization with your healthcare supplier. People may have diverse medical conditions that coincide with a specific agony issue, and that may influence the decision and the conveyance technique for cannabis. All included ought not just comprehend the various sorts (strains) of medical grade cannabis that exists, yet in addition the conveyance frameworks accessible.

Also, you have to know the run of the mill impacts of medical marijuana just as reactions that could happen. For instance, somebody with past mind damage posed me a keen inquiry, *will cannabis fry my cerebrum?* Another individual living with asthma, communicated worries about cannabis impact on the lung whenever he breathed in through vaping. Concerns like these will affect your choice how to choose, how to use, or regardless of whether to use. How about we talk about these issues. As a matter of first importance, there is no single, clear answer at the present time. As expressed in a past blog, Pot for Pain Relief? What the Research Gurus Say , research discoveries are constrained, however encouraging. Getting your work done is basic.

Instructions To Choose

As indicated by Marijuanadoctors.com, there are a great many strains of cannabis that exist. Most fall into three classes: indica, sativa and half breed. There are others, for example, cannabis ruderalis and modern hemp; which are not very much considered.

Indica: All the more steadying, arrives in an assortment of flavors and contains significant levels of pitch. Can come in unadulterated and mixed structures. Indica strains are developed in harsher atmospheres like the center east, Northern Africa, and Nepal. Normally recommended for the accompanying conditions:

- Help with discomfort
- Uneasiness and Stress Disorders
- Seizure Disorders
- Muscle Spasms

Sativa: All the more animating and invigorating, it may manufacture innovativeness. It furthermore comes in combination of fruity-sweet to characteristic flavors. Sativa is created in the Far East, South America and Mexico. Used, anyway not by and large prescribed, for the going with conditions:

- Distress
- Improved focus and ingenuity
- Perspective Elevation
- A resting issue

Note: Pure sativa can start sporadic heartbeats and doubt.

Half and half: regularly a mix of indica and sativa; strain's are mixed for positive properties and favored characteristics. Makers (similarly called reproducers) are resolved in making a collection to address the perfect effects both by recreational and medical purchasers.

Cross breed: Ordinarily a blend of indica and sativa; strain's are blended for positive properties and favored attributes. Cultivators (additionally called raisers) are tenacious in making an assortment to address the ideal impacts both by recreational and medical purchasers. Hence, most medical cannabis is cross breed, which means crossovers are normally a blend of seeds from various nations worldwide where marijuana can effectively develop. Cross breed can be used for:

- Hoisting Mood
- Invigorating Activities and Productivity
- Decline social nervousness
- Improve inspiration
- Overcome social nervousness

- Persuade your psyche

- Decline weakness

- Help with discomfort

- Lift sorrow

- Improve hunger

- Decline nausea and improve assimilation

Mixture: Commonly a blend of indica and sativa; strain's are blended for positive properties and favored qualities. Cultivators (likewise called reproducers) are determined in making an assortment to address the ideal impacts both by recreational and medical customers.

In this way, most medical cannabis is half and half, which means crossovers are ordinarily a mix of seeds from various nations worldwide where marijuana can effectively develop. Half breeds can be used for:

- Lifting Mood

- Stimulating Activities and Productivity

- Diminishing social nervousness

- Improve inspiration

- Vanquish social nervousness

- Propel your psyche

- Diminishing weakness

- Relief from discomfort

- Lift melancholy

- Improve craving

- Reduction nausea and improve processing

Nod of seeds from different countries worldwide where marijuana can viably create. Half breeds can be used for:

- Raising Mood

- Stimulating Activities and Productivity

- Reducing social pressure

- Improve motivation

- Beat social pressure

- Motivate your mind

- Reduction exhaustion

- Help with inconvenience

- Lift misery

- Improve hunger

- Reduction nausea and improve handling

Tranquilizer

Strains can be used in mix, for example, with misery or exhaustion. Sativa could be suggested for daytime use. For sleep deprivation and agony, Indica may be recommended to be used around evening time. These strains regularly have one of kind names, for example,

Lemon Haze (Sativa): Happy, euphoric and elevating; assists with tension, torment, absence of craving

Jack Herer (Sativa): Cerebral, vigorous and innovative; assists with despondency, weariness, nausea

Blue Dream (Hybrid): Relaxed, tired, torment alleviating and social; assists with cerebral pains, aggravation, muscle fits

Blue God (Indica): Pain alleviation, expanded craving and a casual state; assists with sleep deprivation, stress, torment.

Medical quality stains ought to contain more CBD (cannabidiol), which has remedial impacts, than THC (tetrahydocannibidiol); THC has psychoactive properties which causes the *high* favored by recreational users.

Step By Step Instructions To Use

Smoking: Smoking is the most outstanding conveyance framework, where dried leaves are either folded into little cigarettes (doobie, joint, reefer), or put in a pipe or bong (water pipe), which is lit and smoke is breathed in.

Advantages: Smoking gives quick acting alleviation from torment, nausea or different side effects, the guideline of dosing is simple, lower cost and little requirement for leaf preparing in this way progressively unadulterated.

Disadvantages: Smoking is not the best choice on the off chance that you have asthma, visit respiratory sicknesses, incessant bronchitis, COPD or lung malignant growth. Additionally, it must be said that numerous healthcare suppliers are not for empowering breathing in smoke into the lungs in any capacity whatsoever. Tar and other waste products breathed in into the lungs and throat, can aggravate and dry the defensive mucous layers, expanding the danger of disease. Also, the smell of cannabis smoke is observable and thought about hostile to a few.

Disintegrating or *vaping* is a prevalent method for breathing in cannabis (just as tobacco):

This includes preheating a disintegrating gadget to suggested temperature, embeddings a modest quantity of cannabis bloom into the *vape* and afterward breathing in.

Advantages: disintegrating cannabis gives moment alleviation (like smoking), remember the time factor required to warmth up the vaporizer. Vaping does not disturb the mucous layers of the throat and lungs as much as smoking.

Disadvantages: Vaping gadgets will in general be expensive; the procedure of vaping for the unpracticed can be testing or cumbersome just as the exceptional impacts for those not certain what is in store. The smell of cannabis smoke is less yet still present.

Edibles: Cannabis is added to common sweet top choices like brownies, treats, confections, dessert, and chewables (like gum). This can be a favored method to ingest for kids and more established grown-ups.

Advantages: edibles are a satisfying method to ingest cannabis, particularly for the individuals who incline toward not to breathe in smoke; no exceptional hardware is required and no smell of smoke is available.

Disadvantages: palatable structures take additional time before the cannabis impact is observable; in this way dosing can be all the more testing. When the impact is felt it very well may be more extreme than foreseen. Like any oral medicine, it ought to be kept far from small kids and pets to avoid unplanned ingestion.

Tinctures: Type of cannabis disintegrated in liquor that can be set on the skin or taken by mouth by putting drops under the tongue or adding to a cup of hot refreshment; once in a while comes in splash structure. Requires progressive dosing to abstain from taking excessively, too early (dependable guideline: start low, go moderate)

Advantages: quicker acting than edibles, yet more slow than breathed in; mellow taste; simple to manage or take.

Disadvantages: less exorbitant when little portions required, all the more expensive with higher dosing necessities.

Oils/Concentrates: concentrates of cannabis infused into cooking oils, like olive oil or coconut oil, which is then cooked into nourishments.

Advantages: Can be effectively be added to most loved dinners and treats; can be used with people, similar to those with Alzheimers, who cannot comprehend its use or would oppose taking different types of cannabis or drugs of any sort.

Disadvantages: Like edibles.

Topicals: Salves, creams or fixes applied to the skin; most usually used for agony issue, where the topical can be set over the region of torment, for example, joint inflammation, fibromyalgia (trigger focuses) and musculoskeletal torment.

Advantages: Moisturizers/creams give quick beginning, and fleeting help contrasted with patches that give more slow beginning yet longer alleviation. A few people use a mix of creams/salves and fix application to amplify beginning and length of impact.

Disadvantages: Neighborhood hypersensitive response to fix glue/material or restricting specialist in cream/salve has been accounted for.

Different structures (less regularly used): Suppositories, capsules, squeezing (cannabis infused beverages), eating plant leaves.

Much the same as any help with discomfort choice, cannabis may fill in as a key segment of one individual's torment toolbox and not for another. It is definitely not a one size fits all treatment alternative. This is a choice that ought to be talked about with your healthcare supplier before searching out an authorized marijuana prescriber and gadget. On the off chance that you are as of now taking narcotics for relief from discomfort, see whether you will be required to decrease before cannabis is begun. Before having a talking about with your healthcare supplier, be certain you have gotten your work done.

Check laws and guidelines on medical marijuana in your state and network as they differ. Some different territories to address are:

Will medical marijuana influence your capacity to work and perform anticipated obligations?

Will your activity be secure or is there a danger of employment misfortune if medical marijuana is legitimately recommended?

Is there a danger of losing business related trusted status because of medical marijuana use?

What do you have to know whether you traverse state lines or outside the U.S. while utilizing medical marijuana?

What are the buying rules and confinements in the event that you travel for business or diversion out of state or outside the U.S?

CANNABIS PHENOTYPE AND GENOTYPE

In some cases you discover a cannabis strain so great, you can't resist the urge to return to the experience each time the open door presents itself. One day you may be amazed to find another cluster of Blue Dream looks in no way like the one you last attempted: what was before a lance formed blossom currently resembles a thick bulb of precious stone trichomes. It is a similar strain, so, what is with the fluctuation?

Two things impact the basic development of some random cannabis plant: hereditary qualities and condition.

The plant's hereditary cosmetics, additionally called a genotype, goes about as an outline for development: it permits a range of physical conceivable outcomes, yet it is dependent upon the earth to prompt these attributes. The physical articulation of a genotype is alluded to as a phenotype, which is just characterized as the characteristics that nature hauls out from the plant's hereditary code. Everything from shading, shape, smell, and gum production are influenced by the earth.

This manual for cannabis hereditary qualities will help you through the development of the cannabis plant, from its antique beginnings through the present modern development. Before its finish, you will comprehend that there are in fact characterizing attributes for each strain, yet each plant is as extraordinary as a snowflake as it interestingly communicates qualities as indicated by its nursery condition.

The Earliest Cannabis Species

Cannabis is an antiquated plant with roots everywhere throughout the world. The soonest species are thought to have developed in the bumpy Hindu Kush area of Pakistan, while others later multiplied in tropical atmospheres. These most punctual assortments, called landrace strains, are viewed as the precious stones of cannabis hereditary qualities. A large number of long stretches of adjustment enabled these strains to express their absolute best qualities for a particular geological area. These territories are what raisers like DJ Short call *sweet spots*.

Our short, sap overwhelming indicas populated scopes between thirty to fifty degrees, while the tall, slow-developing sativas normally estate in central areas around thirty degrees scope. These assorted natural surroundings adapted a bright cluster of cannabis assortments, each with its very own long-standing history.

Cannabis in the Great Indoors

Cannabis reproducing took a significant turn starting during the 1970s and 80s when government hostile to cannabis opinions crested, driving development from nature to underground. Indoor gardens, raised by soil, electric lights, and hydroponic frameworks, produce a main part of the cannabis found in the market today. While little uncertainty astonishingly developed strains have been developed inside, specialists will concur that the conventional, unnatural condition can just bring out such a large amount of the plant's potential.

Narrowing decent variety significantly further, producers during this time were fundamentally propelled by THC substance and specifically picked this trademark over other significant concoction constituents like CBD. Disregarding this lost lavishness, we see incredible fluctuation in the plant's phenotypic articulation: supplements, temperature, the sum and point of light, soil type, photoperiod length, time of gather, and the separation between the plant and light source are among the numerous conditions that influence the plant's qualities. Certain conditions may cajole sativa-or indica-like characteristics, so as much as we love arranging strains here at Leafly, we need to recognize that a strain's qualities are not really set in hereditary stone.

The Age of Hybridization

Connected at the hip with the indoor develop transformation came hybridized strains, an intermixing of worldwide indigenous assortments. This is the point at which the sativa met the indica, starting a consistently spreading tree of hybrid posterity. Cultivators appreciated indicas for their pitch covered buds and short blooming periods, the two of which are desired characteristics for business production.

In the event that we consider indicas and sativas as falling on furthest edges of the hereditary range, it gets conceivable to envision the extent of phenotypic articulation. Take Blue Dream for instance: a cross between the indica Blueberry and sativa Haze, Blue Dream may think about attributes anyplace the range between its folks, contingent upon how it was raised. This is the reason we may now and then observe an indica-like phenotype of Blue Dream when we expect a sativa. That is not to say strains are eccentric hereditary special cases; rather, we just shouldn't be astounded when a strain doesn't fit splendidly inside an unmitigated box. Once more, it is conceivable to coax sativa or indica qualities with explicit conditions in a controlled nursery.

Because of hybridization, we have a for all intents and purposes boundless choice of strains to choose from and even energetic strain gatherers will consistently have new hybrids to pursue. Expert focused cultivators may grieve the loss of unique cannabis hereditary qualities, however many still commit themselves to their restoration. Not exclusively would their recovery make for a more extravagant recreational market, *antiquated* strains could tremendously affect cannabis as medicine. We trust that as political obstructions fall over like dominoes, the agricultural craft of cannabis development will have the option to sprout all inclusive by and by.

Really, cannabis rearing is turning out to be more science than workmanship, the impacts of which can be used for everything from torment management to fiber making. Tragically, preclusion has carried with it no shortage of negative symptoms, including an absence of logical examination and distribution about the plant. Simultaneously, the more we find out about cannabis, the more we're starting to understand that things we once thought to be genuine are in reality bogus. A raiser keen on creating a plant with smooth impacts, for instance, may cross two assortments ordinarily alluded to as *indicas*, just to locate those *two indicas* contain much more THC than they would have suspected.

Behind these misinterpretations is a basic idea that we've just barely started examining in cannabis: hereditary qualities. In this post, we'll spread some significant ideas and learnings in cannabis hereditary qualities and see how understanding cannabis hereditary qualities can assume a basic job in reproducing that ideal cultivar.

The Basics: Debunking the Indica versus Sativa Binary

The best spot to begin is with the manner in which the vast majority think with regards to arranging cannabis: indica and sativa. Regular terminology places these ordered groupings into a sort of parallel: *sativa* assortments are restricted leafed, tall, lean, and invigorating, while *indica* assortments are expansive leaf, short, ragged and calming.

As we test and find out about these assortments, in any case, we are discovering that the inverse can be valid: tight leaf assortments regularly have calming impacts and wide leaf assortments can be invigorating. So, how would you know what an assortment is or what it does? Extremely, the best way to appropriately characterize assortments is to know the chemotype, the cannabinoid and terpene profile, alongside the genotype, its one of kind hereditary cosmetics.

Genotype Versus Phenotypes

Genotype depends on the DNA of a living being. Cannabis is diploid, implying that it acquires two duplicates of every quality, one duplicate from each parent. Consequently, the genotype for a quality of intrigue depends on the blend of the two duplicates.

Phenotypes are the noticeable qualities or attributes of a plant that are dictated by genotype and physical condition (counting however not restricted to temperature, moistness, and development rehearses). A few phenotypes, like leaf shape and bloom shading can be seen, though others, for example, the chemotype of a plant (the concoction phenotype, similar to terpene profile and cannabinoid strength) must be estimated.

Cannabis hereditary qualities work likewise: one parent plant might be expansive leafed with low degrees of THC, while the other is thin leafed with significant levels of THC. Their youngsters (the seeds) will contain hereditary qualities from the two guardians, and just a portion of those characteristics will communicate when the plant really develops. This is the reason the morphology of the plant, or the manner in which it looks is definitely not an adequate sign of its synthetic substance. Nor, in any case, is a hereditary quality, even clones of precisely the same plant may convey what needs be contrastingly relying upon how they are developed. For instance, a clone raised in an indoor developing office may deliver diverse morphology and chemotype levels than one become outside. Thus, indistinguishable twins may not be superbly indistinguishable: one might be brought into the world with a mole on their cheek, or they may create various physiologies on the off chance that they experience childhood in various situations or have diverse eating and exercise propensities. Along these lines, even precisely the same genotype can deliver various phenotypes.

Characterizing Cannabis sativa

Understanding that indica and sativa are not really a paired and that there is, rather, a universe of hereditary assorted variety, prompts a truly significant inquiry: what, at that point, is Cannabis sativa? Are there genuinely different cannabis species?

Here is where hereditary qualities can assist us with finding the appropriate response: through looking at DNA between a large number of tests, we can start to reveal some insight into the connections between various cultivars of cannabis, just as the species limit.

CANNABIS STRAINS

Strains Of Cannabis – Indica Versus Sativa Versus Hybrid

Alright, so now we should discuss these various strains of weed, where they originate from, the distinction between the plants and their development, and what their consequences for the human body are.

Sources

The words Indica and Sativa were both acquainted in the eighteenth century with depict the two fundamental kinds of cannabis strains. These are cannabis Indica and cannabis Sativa.The term cannabis Indica was instituted by Jean-Baptiste Lamarck, and this was initially used to portray marijuana for the most part found in India which is high in psychoactive properties, where it was developed and gathered basically for fiber, seeds, and the production of hashish (increasingly here on the distinction among hash and weed). The term cannabis Sativa was authored via Carl Linneaus and was initially used to depict marijuana plants developed in Europe and Western Asia, where it was collected fundamentally for fiber and seeds, yet additionally for its different properties. Since the eighteenth century, there have been numerous newfound and hereditarily adjusted strains of marijuana, with hybrid strains, which are goes among Sativa and Indica, not being made until numerous years after the fact.

Consequences for The Body

Something which is critical to note with regards to the contrasts between Sativa, Indica, and hybrid weed strains is that they easily affect the human body. At the end of the day, these three fundamental sorts of weed impact you in various manners when smoked, disintegrated, or eaten.

Cannabis Indica is for the most part an evening weed and is best smoked or eaten when you have dealt with the entirety of your obligations regarding the day. Indica strains are known for the accompanying impacts on the human body:

- Extraordinary for mental unwinding.

- Assists with muscle unwinding.

- Diminishes sickness.

- Helps increment hunger.

- Helps decline intense and serious agony.

- Expands dopamine – alleviates pressure and discouragement.

- Causes supposed love *seat lock* – best for evening use.

Then again, cannabis Sativa is generally a greater amount of an invigorating kind of marijuana which most would consider best for daytime use. The impacts of cannabis Sativa on the human body incorporate the accompanying:

- Incredible for assuaging uneasiness.

- Useful for calming pressure.

- Helps increment serotonin – controls state of mind.

- Builds innovativeness and center, in a specific way.

- Functions admirably for constant agony.

- Will in general be genuinely invigorating - useful for daytime use.

- Remember that hybrid cannabis strains, due to being a blend of Sativa and Indica strains, can contain a specific level of these properties.

This will rely upon the level of the kinds of weed included when making the Hybrid strains. A few cross breeds can be completely adjusted among Indica and Sativa, some can be Indica prevailing, and some can be Sativa predominant.

Plant Appearance and Growth

Something different which is important here is that Sativa and Indica strains appear to be unique when they are being developed. At the end of the day, Indica weed plants appear to be unique from Sativa weed plants, and they have somewhat extraordinary development cycle qualities as well. Remember that crossover marijuana strains can extraordinarily vary as far as the plant appearance and development qualities, and it truly depends whether the half breed is a Sativa prevailing, Indica predominant, or a decent strain.

The appearance and development attributes of cannabis Sativa plants incorporate the accompanying:

Cannabis Sativa plants will in general be very tall with genuinely limited leaves. These plants will in general have a genuinely long blossoming cycle, so they take somewhat long to develop and prepare for collect Cannabis Sativa plants are typically most appropriate for development in warm atmospheres which have a long developing season.

The appearance and development qualities of cannabis Indica plants incorporate the accompanying:

Cannabis Indica plants will in general be shorter in stature and bushier than Sativa plants, and have a lot more extensive leaves. Cannabis Indica plants have a shorter blossoming cycle than Sativa plants, by as much as two or three weeks, and in this manner are snappier to develop and get the chance to reap. Cannabis Indica plants are most appropriate for marginally cooler atmospheres with to some degree shorter developing seasons.

DIFFERENCE BETWEEN THC AND CBD STRAINS

Something that is likewise imperative to note here is the contrast among CBD and THC. What you cannot deny is that marijuana contains something known as cannabinoids. The weed plant has many synthetic substances in it. The primary segments which cause the real and mental impacts are terpenes and cannabinoids. The two principle and most basic cannabinoids are THC and CBD, and they can have altogether different consequences for the body and psyche.

THC Dominant Marijuana Strains

THC represents Tetrahydrocannabinol. These are the strains which are typically picked by individuals who need an unwinding and calming strain for evening use. They are extraordinary for treating extreme agony, an absence of hunger, sickness, tension, gloom, and that's only the tip of the iceberg. This is the sort of weed that gives you a solid and euphoric head high, will in general make you genuinely drained, and it causes hunger too. This is the sort of weed that gives you the munchies.

CBD Dominant Marijuana Strains

CBD represents cannabidiol. This is really a non-inebriating compound. As such, it does not create an euphoric head high. It as a rule does not cause tiredness or yearning, in any event on the off chance that you just smoke a touch of it. This is a decent strain to go with to ease ceaseless torment, to move innovativeness, to diminish aggravation, and that is only the tip of the iceberg. It's a decent decision to go with in the event that you need help from different side effects, however don't need that yearning actuating, love seat locking head high. Something significant here is that there is a misguided judgment that CBD overwhelming strains are really invigorating. People, Sativa Is not a similar thing as a Red Bull or some espresso. It simply does not work that way. While CBD overwhelming strains won't make you as worn out, or cause you to wear out as awful as Indica substantial strains, they will inevitably still make you somewhat drained, simply less so than Indica.

Adjusted CBD and THC Marijuana Strains

Marijuana strains which contain a parity of THC and CBD is a decision which numerous individuals will in general go with. These strains will in general produce a mellow to respectably euphoric head high, a touch of appetite, and are really useful for sleep deprivation, while they additionally contain a specific measure of manifestation help. This truly relies upon the harmony among THC and CBD, and can change incredibly starting with one strain then onto the next.

Sativa Versus Indica And CBD Versus THC – A Common Misconception Cannabis Plant Appearance

What is entrancing to note is that for a long time, it was acknowledged that most Indica strains contain more CBD than THC, and that Sativa strains contained more THC than CBD. Regardless, this is not commonly the circumstance in any way shape or form. As a rule, if you somehow happened to inspect hundred marijuana strains, the outcome ought to be that Indica strains by and large contain all the more calming THC, while most Sativa strains contain more CBD. This is significant on the grounds that this has been an extremely huge misguided judgment for quite a while. Despite that fact, what you likewise need to know is that the profiles of Indica, Sativa, and hybrid strains have changed and broadened after some time.

Presently, it is never again exact to state one way or the other. Some Indica strains may be truly elevated in CBD or THC, however not the other, or both, and this goes for Sativa and hybrid strains as well. In spite of the fact that the Indica, Sativa, and hybrid characterizations still stay famous and broadly utilized today, they are not constantly exact regarding educating the shopper regarding the genuine THC and CBD includes in them. This is the reason you have to investigate every individual strain before settling on an acquiring choice.

A Note On Terpenes

As we referenced over, another of the fundamental mixes found in all marijuana strains are terpenes. In the event that you did not have the foggiest idea, terpenes are a kind of sweet-smelling compound created by most leafy foods, and indeed, marijuana is a blooming plant.

You will discover terpenes contained in numerous sweet-smelling blossoms, lavender, citrus organic products, peppers, and indeed, cannabis as well. Terpenes are the principle contributing element to that fruity, fancy, citrusy, berry-like, and numerous different aromas and tastes which your strain of marijuana may highlight. Various strains of weed contain various terpenes, and there are a wide range of sorts of terpenes to go around.

There are a couple of extremely regular terpenes found in marijuana. One of these is linalool, which is known to be unwinding. Another regular terpene found in cannabis is pinene, which highlights a greater amount of a cautioning property. Be that as it may, the truth is that making sense of which terpenes cause which impacts is truly difficult to measure. None the less, it merits inspecting the most well-known terpenes found in marijuana;

- **Alpha Pinene** – This terpene scents like pine or pine needles, it will in general increment sharpness and memory maintenance, and can be utilized for treating asthma, agony, irritation, and nervousness.

- **Myrcene** – This terpene has a musky, natural, and home grown like smell, and regularly scents like cloves or cardamom. Mycrene will in general have an unwinding, quieting, and lounge chair locking impact. It is a decent enemy of oxidant, it assists with a sleeping disorder, agony, and irritation.

- **Limonene** – This terpene has a very citrusy smell and flavor, and it hoists your state of mind and helps with pressure alleviation. It tends to be utilized to treat uneasiness, stress, gloom, irritation, and agony.

- **Caryophyllene** – This terpene has a zesty and peppery smell and taste, regularly woody too. This is an extraordinary terpene for stress alleviation and is regularly known to help with agony, tension, and gloom.

- **Linalool** – This terpene has an extremely extravagant smell and taste. It has the impacts of sedation and mind-set improvement. It very well may be utilized to help treat sleep deprivation, torment, melancholy, tension, stress, and irritation.

- **Humulene** – This terpene has a hoppy, natural, and woody flavor. It's best known for having calming properties.

- **Ocimene** – Ocimene is a terpene which has a sweet, woody, and natural like smell and flavor. It is outstanding for having hostile to septic, against contagious, and against viral properties, and it is referred to as a decongestant too.

- **Terpinolene** – This terpene has a flower, piney, and home grown aroma and flavor. It is unwinding, it fills in as an enemy of oxidant, and is soothing in nature.

Most popular strains of cannabis

Here, we just want to list some of the most popular and widely purchased strains of Cannabis in all 3 categories, Sativa, Indica, and hybrid. These strains are definitely worth trying out.

Sativa:

- Acapulco Gold

- Allen Wrench

- Amnesia

- Chocolope

- Cinex

- Dirty Girl

- Durban Poison

- Ghost Train Haze

- Grapefruit

- Green Crack

- Harlequin

- Sweet Skunk

- Jack Herer

- Kali Mist

- Maui Wowie

- Purple Haze

- Sour Diesel

- Lemon Haze

- Silver Haze

Indica:

- Afghani

- Blueberry

- Bubba Kush

- G13

- Granddaddy Purple

- Green Ape

- Hindu Kush

- Lavender

- Master Kush

- Northern Lights

- Presidential OG

- Purple Urkle

Hybrid:

- ACDC

- Ak-47

- Banana OG

- Blue Dream

- Catatonic

- Chernobyl

- Cherry Pie

- Cinderella 99

- Double Dream

- Dutch Treat

- Fruity Pebbles

- Gelato

- Jillybean

- Juicy Fruit

- Larry OG

- Lodi Dodi

- Mango Kush

- OG Kush

- Permafrost

- Pineapple Express

- Pink Kush

- Snoop's Dream

- Sour Tsunami

- Space Queen

- Tahoe OG

- Trainwreck

- UK Cheese

- White Fire OG

- White Widow

Picking The Right Cannabis Strain For You

Presently you know pretty much everything there is to think about the different strains and sorts of weed. Allows simply emphasize some central matters of center with regards to picking the correct sort of marijuana for you. What would you like to escape your smoking, disintegrating, or edibles experience? Do you need help with discomfort, tension and sorrow management? Do you need something to make you hungry, do you experience the ill effects of sleep deprivation? On the off chance that you are utilizing marijuana for medical conditions, you have to pick the correct strain, with the best possible CBD and THC content for the activity.

What scents and smells do you like? Indeed, this is alluding to the terpenes. You may like weed that is greater fruity, woody, nutty, natural, citrusy, or whatever else. Consider the terpene and flavor profile of the marijuana strain being referred to before settling on a decision. It is safe to say that you are smoking, vaping, or eating edibles during the day or around evening time? As a rule, Sativa won't make you as worn out or ravenous as Indica strains as well, something essential to remember whether you plan on being dynamic during the day or need a decent night's rest. Keep in mind that THC is the thing that creates an euphoric head high, while CBD generally does not deliver a lot of a high by any means. CBD is best for side effect help, while THC is incredible for making you feel high.

Conceivable Side Effects Of THC Marijuana Dominant Strains

Before we wrap up for the afternoon, something you should know is that for certain individuals, strains which are exceptionally overwhelming in THC can cause some symptoms. Presently, this is definitely not a slam dunk, as everyone responds in an unexpected way. Sadly, this is a preliminary by blunder sort of thing, and you won't ever truly know how you will respond to THC substantial weed until you attempt it for yourself. Notwithstanding, basically a mess of THC can possibly create some entirely serious reactions in individuals, and truly, there are individuals who are adversely affected by it. On the off chance that you need tension and help with discomfort, however can not deal with a great deal of THC, you should go with a CBD overwhelming strain, or possibly one that is well-adjusted between the two.

A portion of the conceivable reactions of THC substantial marijuana strains incorporate the accompanying:

- Tension

- Melancholy

- Suspicion (One of the most widely recognized reactions in numerous individuals)

- Outrageous laziness – love seat lock

- Cerebral pains

- Tipsiness

- Wooziness

- Dry and irritated eyes

Presently you should know essentially everything about the contrasts between Indica, Sativa, and hybrid marijuana strains. To individuals who are not customary cannabis clients, this may sound somewhat trifling. Be that as it may, regardless of anything else, there are some huge contrasts between the principle strains and sorts of weed. Realizing the distinctions will assist you with picking the correct one dependent on what sort of impacts and results you are hoping to accomplish.

GREENHOUSE CULTIVATION OF CANNABIS FOR SEEDS USED IN PRODUCTION OF CANNABIS PHARMACY OIL

With any greenhouse structure, it is imperative to remember the end reason directly from the beginning. Greenhouses are worked to give your yield, whatever it is, with the perfect developing condition. On the off chance that you are developing annuals or perennials you may need to assemble some adaptability in your greenhouse structure to oblige various plants with various climatic needs. On the off chance that you are just developing tomatoes, your greenhouse can be structured worked to concentrate altogether on boosting production efficiencies and yield of that plant.

Marijuana is a controlled substance, so expecting you have paid some dues to be granted one of the pined for cultivation licenses, it is far-fetched that your marijuana greenhouse will develop any plants outside the cannabis family. So for developing marijuana plants, you need to concentrate on the perfect condition for cannabis.

The four Stages of Growth for Cannabis Production Affect How You Zone Your Greenhouse

- Zone 1: Marijuana mother plants

- Zone 2: Marijuana clones (cuttings)

- Zone 3: Marijuana in the vegetative stage

- Zone 4: Marijuana in the bloom stage

Plan for Expansion from the Start

On the off chance that you are as of now developing harvests effectively in a greenhouse, it is anything but difficult to concentrate your cannabis business energies on the yield developing side. Be that as it may, dismissing this all in all new business with various clients and distinctive circulation directs will get you in a tough situation. Start your cannabis greenhouse measured for your not so distant future client requests yet in view of adaptability to suit your more drawn out term business objectives. We work with cultivators everywhere throughout the world structuring greenhouses for different stage extension plans. Some additional time toward the start can spare you long stretches of migraines and extra expenses not far off.

Parity Production Efficiencies

Marijuana producers are accustomed to developing in littler spaces than most business cultivators. Greenhouse structures and modern plant developing innovation offer huge production advantages contrasted with run of the mill indoor developing. Be that as it may, where huge zones increment production productivity, they additionally increment harvest chance from ailment or pervasion spreading. At the point when you consider the financial estimation of your marijuana crop, and perhaps the medical basic of giving reliable medicine to your patients, there is a sensible tradeoff between production scale zones and detachment portioning.

Zone division can without much of a stretch be accomplished with inside peak dividers and sidewalls, an appropriately structured greenhouse warming and cooling framework and great natural controls. Power outage blinds (otherwise called light hardship screens), water system, and fertigation frameworks are altogether structured by greenhouse industry specialists to be midway controlled for numerous zones.

Building the Ideal Environment

- **Geographic area:** I can not overemphasize the significance of this point. Not every greenhouse maker or cannabis developing specialists have involvement with various land areas. Numerous individuals will attempt to sell you the greenhouse that has been effective in Colorado, however in the event that you are in Southern California, Puerto Rico, or Alaska, the greenhouse you need will be altogether different. You are outside temperature vacillations, wind speeds, stickiness levels, snow loads, and light levels all factor into what gear and the style of structure that is best for you and your yield.

- **Inside greenhouse temperature:** Cannabis like numerous harvests likes various temperatures at various stages of development. As a speculation you need your greenhouse temperatures between 65 to 85° F. Your greenhouse warming and cooling frameworks need to consider the temperature needs and controls for each zone. Unpracticed experts may disclose to you that you don't require as a lot of warming on the grounds that the lights produce a great deal of warmth, yet as you will find in the segments underneath, cannabis ordinarily needs just eighteen or twelve hours of light, so your coldest evening time temperatures will in any case commonly have no lights on by any stretch of the imagination.

- **Overseeing stickiness inside a cannabis greenhouse:** We as a whole know the impacts stickiness has on plants. To an extreme, and you welcome illness, excessively little and you dry out the plant and prevent development. Similarly as with any harvest, knowing the dampness that the plant flourishes in is significant when planning a greenhouse. While cannabis in the vegetative stage really loves a higher moistness level, it lean towards lower stickiness when in blossom. Greenhouse producers who comprehend this can assist you with building adaptability into your greenhouse structures. There are a few dehumidification units available, and for zones requiring the capacity to include dampness moistening frameworks can be included into the greenhouse structure.

- **Ventilation proposals for greenhouses tie into temperature and moistness needs:** Greenhouse ventilation separates into two fundamental classifications: 1) common ventilation spreads rooftop vents, sidewall vents and rollup sides, and 2) constrained air ventilation requires mechanical frameworks like fumes fans, and in some cases cooling cushions. Kindly note that cooling cushions are not a decent choice for high dampness districts. Notwithstanding ventilation to expel tourist from inside the greenhouse, most greenhouse cultivators put wind stream fans inside the greenhouse to flow air development which is useful for keeping healthy plants. Greenhouse makers can furnish you with a greenhouse plan design demonstrating fan areas that streamline wind stream coverage.

- **Altering lighting levels will build yields in a cannabis greenhouse**: Perhaps the greatest advantage that greenhouse developing ideas over indoor developing is that greenhouse plants profit by common daylight. Not exclusively does daylight normally give the plants what they have to develop, it does not cost the cultivator any cash to control. Having said that, when cannabis is in the vegetative state it performs best with around eighteen hours of light. Therefore we prescribe greenhouse cultivators incorporate supplemental lighting in their cannabis greenhouse arrangement. Ensure your greenhouse lighting plans fulfill all year production on the off chance that you need to upgrade yields.

- **Blossoming cannabis needs power outage.** While the vegetative stage appreciates more prominent light levels, for blooming longer times of murkiness are wanted. Guaranteeing twelve hours of continuous murkiness inside your greenhouse will constrain the marijuana plants to bloom as per your production plan. This is best accomplished by using power outage window ornament innovation, otherwise called light hardship in the marijuana business. Power outage has been ordinarily utilized in production greenhouses for quite a long time for poinsettias, kalanchoes, mums and other crops that profit by photoperiod changes. Power outage blinds can cover level rooftop zones running bracket to support on canal associated greenhouses, or they can be slanted to pursue the rooftop line of detached greenhouses. Make sure to cover sidewalls and entryway openings, and at GGS we give light traps to debilitate fans too.

- **Cannabis plants flourish with CO2 advancement:** On the off chance that you are utilizing a high temp water warming framework CO_2 can be pulled off the boiler. In different cases you may wish to utilize fluid CO_2 to portion your cannabis crop. This is a zone best examined with greenhouse warming specialists like our sister organization Niagrow Systems. Extra contemplations incorporate associating your greenhouse to distribution center and office offices for bundling, delivery, and other bolster capacities. There are other exceptional necessities for cannabis that you won't have experienced with run of the mill plant crops, for example, drying rooms and vaults. Work with an organization that has the mastery to support you.

- **Supplement:** Supplements are taken up from the soil by roots. Supplement soil corrections (composts) are included when the soil supplements are drained. Manures can be compound or natural, fluid or powder, and as a rule contain a blend of fixings. Business composts indicate the degrees of NPK (nitrogen, phosphorus, and potassium). When all is said in done, cannabis needs more N than P and K during all life stages. The nearness of auxiliary supplements (calcium, magnesium, sulfur) is suggested. Micronutrients (for example iron, boron, chlorine, manganese, copper, zinc, molybdenum) infrequently show as insufficiencies. Since cannabis' supplement needs differ generally relying upon the assortment, they are typically dictated by experimentation and manures are applied sparingly to abstain from consuming the plant.

Picking Your Perfect Cannabis Seed for Production

Concerning gathering, one of the most empowering things you can choose to accumulate are cannabis seeds. These questionable little beans are one of the most genetically planned normal products available, likely only to some degree behind roses. The astonishing qualities alongside the sheer number of various strains of seed accessible make them one of the most fascinating and most overwhelming accumulations to begin. One of the missions a few gatherers embrace is to attempt to locate their ideal cannabis seed. Each unique strain holds an alternate arrangement of ascribes which will join to give you the ideal seed that matches your taste.

THC: THC means *Tetrahydrocannabinol.* This is the principle psychoactive part found in a completely developed cannabis plant and when you search for seeds you will see the THC rate recorded. While your seeds won't contain any genuine THC, each strain has been intended to dependably deliver a plant that will have this degree of THC. In the event that you are fortunate enough to live in a nation where developing cannabis is legitimate you will have the option to test it out. On the off chance that you are not, you should manage with your ideal seed having the capacity to deliver certain degrees of THC.

Yield: Another thing you may get a kick out of the chance to think about your cannabis seed is how a lot of cannabis it could make on the off chance that it were lawful to develop it. Yield is typically estimated in grams and is worked out by the normal yield found by the reproducer. In the event that you like to realize your seed could deliver a high return this is a credit you may get a kick out of the chance to take a gander at.

Strain: Choosing a strain is not just about the imperative measurements however. You find genuinely comparative THC and yield levels on various cannabis seeds so you have to pick a strain you like. A respectable technique to do this is to look at ones that have won bona fide distinctions for quality. The most regarded of which is certainly the High Times Cannabis Cup. Consistently they judge what seed bank and what individual cannabis seed is the best of the year. Feminized seeds are apparently the most de rigueur at the present time.

PRODUCTION OF CANNABIS PHARMACY OIL

Nowadays, CBD oil business is on the ascent. Actually, the market will appreciate fast development as there is a great deal of interest for the product. A couple of individuals do not have the foggiest thought regarding the wellspring of the oil. Everything considered, CBD is short for Cannabidiol. Essentially, the oil is removed from a plant and is helpful for individuals with stress, joint pain and numerous different conditions. On the off chance that you need a couple of strong systems to assist you with beginning and develop your business by selling this oil, you might need to peruse this guide.

- **Register your Business:** First, you have to get a license. As it were, you have to get your business enlisted. This applies regardless of whether you need to open an on the web or physical store. Individuals want to purchase from an enlisted merchant so as to dodge con artists. Purchasing unique products is everybody's worry.

- **Dispatch a Website:** Once you have your business enrolled, your best course of action is to make a site to advertise your products. Ensure your site is average enough. For this, you have to decide on a dependable web designer.

- **Pick a Merchant Processor:** You have to search for a dependable shipper processor. This is significant in the event that you need to get installment for your product deals. While it's legitimate to keep up a CBD oil business, various merchant processors think this kind of business incorporates a huge amount of danger.

- Keep the Law: Once you have picked a trader, your best course of action is to adhere to the government laws. As it were, you should keep the laws identified with the clearance of medical and recreational cannabis products. Thinking about all, you would incline toward not to violate any laws while your business is creating.

- **Run Marketing Campaigns**: Irrespective of the sort of business you run, ensure you find a way to advertise your products. In actuality, marketing is the foundation of any business.

With the correct marketing techniques, you can communicate as the need should arise to a great deal of potential clients. The perfect method for marketing your business is by means of Google promotions, blog entries, and different kinds of advertisements. Beside this, you can utilize the intensity of online networking to arrive at much more clients. In any case, to make your web based life marketing effective, you have to make posts that are locks in. With the help of SEO, you can without quite a bit of a stretch position your site. To answer the request of your customers, you must have a solid customer care organization on your site. Open your Online Store: A straightforward technique for extending your arrangements is to dispatch an online store. You may need to offer a colossal grouping of products through your store. It will be more straightforward for you to build up your customers if you offer a combination of products. All things considered, not all clients like to purchase a similar product. CBD oil is utilized diversely dependent on the kind of condition a patient has.

Production and Extraction Of CBD Oil

Cannabidiol (CBD) is one of numerous normally happening cannabinoid found in the cannabis plant. Both hemp and marijuana can contain CBD, however today CBD products are fundamentally made from hemp. Dissimilar to marijuana which contains a lot of THC, the high prompting compound in cannabis, hemp contains all things considered follow sums.

While there is a developing business sector for smoked hemp blossom, the most well-known approach to devour the gainful phytocompounds is by means of tinctures or containers. So as to be devoured as such, the normally happening mixes in the plant must be separated into oil structure. This oil is then utilized as the essential fixing in these and a lot progressively consumable and topical product.

The technique for extraction and handling of a hemp concentrate can bigly affect the substance, quality, and immaculateness of a given product. In this book, we spread the different techniques for extraction used to make CBD oil from hemp. Continue perusing to find what goes into the making of a CBD product and what sorts of extraction and handling are liked. Hemp has at last been given a definition separate from marijuana. This definition lifts hemp out of the controlled substances act, making the plant and its concentrates lawful. The meaning of hemp is cannabis containing 0.3% or less THC by dry weight. This lawful status and the high-CBD substance of numerous strains has prompted hemp being the essential wellspring of CBD oil extraction for products offered to people in general.

It is conceivable to discover high-CBD products removed from marijuana, yet they are additionally regularly high in THC and in this manner today should be sold as a marijuana product through fitting channels. These products are outside the extent of this book, and any CBD product you find uninhibitedly accessible available to be purchased on the web and in retail locations will be hemp-inferred. This is phenomenal news as it implies there are numerous viable, clean products accessible.

This legitimate endorsement has brought forth an undeniably huge number of cultivators and extractors who look to create the most excellent hemp conceivable. Today you'll discover an abundance of products sourced from naturally developed, non-GMO, local hemp plants.

Comparing CBD Oil Extraction Methods

As we talked about in the introduction, the hemp plant first needs to experience an extraction procedure all together for the plant mixes to be changed into one of the numerous products accessible available today. The general thought of hemp extraction is that a dissolvable is gone through plant material so as to separate out the dynamic mixes in the mass plant materials. The subsequent cannabinoids, terpenes, and other plant mixes like chlorophyll are then gathered as oil and further prepared before advancing into a final result.

The accompanying techniques are for the most part normally used to make the different ranges of CBD oil concentrates found available today. Every strategy conveys impediments and advantages which we spread underneath:

Supercritical CO_2 Extraction-CO_2 extraction is broadly viewed as an incredible technique used to make CBD-rich removes. This extraction technique puts carbon dioxide under high weight while keeping up a low temperature. The gas is changed into a fluid because of the weight and afterward went through the plant material with up to a 90% extraction proficiency. The subsequent concentrates an exceptionally focused, absolutely unadulterated oil separate. This procedure requires costly hardware and experienced administrators. Along these lines, the subsequent oil is regularly more extravagant for the end buyer however empowers the most excellent products to be delivered.

- **Ethanol Extraction**: When contrasted with CO2 extraction, ethanol extraction is a lower-cost technique, yet utilized by numerous organizations available today. Notwithstanding the lower cost, this extraction strategy can at present be utilized to make top notch removes however it might require more mastery and post-extraction handling. This extraction strategy uses a liquor dissolvable - most generally ethanol. Ethanol is 'By and large Regarded as Safe (GRAS)' by the FDA. It is normally utilized as a nourishment additive and added substance found in numerous products at the market. Ethanol is a polar dissolvable which means it will blend in with water and break down water-solvent particles notwithstanding the ideal cannabis mixes. Chlorophyll is one of the intensifies that ethanol will co-remove alongside the cannabinoid filled oil. The outcome is a dim hued oil with a severe and lush flavor.

The chlorophyll can be expelled from the oil utilizing post-extraction sifting techniques, however the procedure can likewise evacuate a portion of the cannabinoids bringing about a lower quality CBD oil product. Some ethanol extractors refer to that the water-solvent part extraction can be alleviated by utilizing cold extraction temperatures. Accepting an accomplished administrator, the aftereffect of this extraction strategy can be truly great, even tantamount to CO_2 extraction in quality. That being stated, with a less experienced extractor, there is more space for blunder and probability for dissolvable tainting or lower quality finished result.

- **Hydrocarbon Extraction**: This early extraction technique was made utilizing a light hydrocarbon dissolvable like to separate cannabis oil. Usually butane, pentane, propane, hexane, isopropyl liquor or CH3)2CO are utilized as solvents. These hydrocarbons have a low boiling point and can be effectively used to extricate CBD oil. This modest and simple technique for extraction accompanies an assortment of issues that make it non-perfect. The subsequent oil generally contains a lower convergence of terpenes and cannabinoids like CBD and a higher centralization of THC. There is likewise risky buildup that can remain that may meddle with safe capacity. This extraction technique demonstrated to be both hazardous a wasteful and is along these lines once in a while utilized by business CBD organizations today.

- **Lipid Extraction**: One of the lesser-utilized extraction techniques is called lipid extraction. This strategy utilizes the fats, or *lipids* in order to assimilate and embody the hemp-delivered mixes. Frequently natural coconut oil is utilized in this extraction procedure. Lipid extraction does not require the utilization of any brutal solvents or CO_2. It is anything but a well known strategy for extraction, however you may discover some boutique organizations utilizing it.

Extra CBD Extract Processing

After a CBD concentrate is made, there are some extra, discretionary steps that are performed to prepare the product for utilization. Actuating by means of Decarboxylation. The normally happening cannabinoids found in the cannabis plant arrive in a corrosive structure including:

- CBDA (Cannabidiolic corrosive)

- THCA (Tetrahydrocannabinolic corrosive)

- CBGA (Cannabigerolic corrosive)

These *crude* cannabinoids must be enacted so as to create the ideal particles. For instance, CBDA must be enacted to deliver CBD. At the point when a low-temperature technique like supercritical CO_2 extraction is utilized, the first corrosive types of the cannabinoids might be created. So as to initiate these cannabinoids and evacuated the corrosive atom, the CBD concentrate experiences a procedure called decarboxylation. Despite the fact that it sounds extravagant, decarboxylation is basically the warming of a concentrate. Through this warming procedure, the corrosive particle is evacuated and the dynamic compound is delivered. Regardless of being less prevalent, the *crude* particles are demonstrating guarantee as they interface with the body uniquely in contrast to the *actuated* or non-corrosive types of these equivalent substances. For instance, THCA is non-psychoactive, while THC is psychoactive. Restricted research and episodic client encounters point to these crude cannabinoid structures giving some interesting helpful benefits.This is driving a few organizations to incorporate the corrosive types of these cannabinoids notwithstanding the enacted non-corrosive structures. All things considered, except if explicitly laid out as a *crude* product, all CBD products available have been decarboxylated to actuate the mixes.

Cleansing by means of Winterization

At the point when the oil concentrate was made utilizing high weight or high temperatures, the extraction procedure pulls a wide scope of unsaturated fats, plant materials, chlorophyll, cannabinoids, and terpenoids from the plant material. For concentrates of this sort, there is a discretionary procedure called winterization which attempts to further filter the concentrate and expel the undesirable parts. The way toward winterizing comprises of totally blending the CBD separate in two-hundred proof liquor and solidifying it medium-term. In the first part of the day the shady blend is prepared for filtration. This procedure is finished by running it through a paper channel into an extraction container. The liquor is expelled from the separated final result through warming until it vanishes. This is made conceivable in light of the fact that the liquor has a lower boiling point than the oil.

How to CBD Isolate is Made?

Since you comprehend CBD extraction, it is opportunity to make things a stride further. Today you'll generally discover single-atom CBD confines. In their most perfect structure, these disengages are a crystalline white powder included 99%+ cannabidiol. All different cannabinoids, terpenes, plant materials, oil, and chlorophyll is evacuated in the production of this powder. All that is left is normally sourced CBD precious stones that convey no smell or flavor. This seclude is made by first extricating oil utilizing one of the techniques we talked about above and afterward winterizing. Next, scientists can utilize short way refining or chromatography disengage the individual mixes in the material, for this situation, cannabidiol. For short way refining, this works similarly as winterization as each compound can be disconnected through their extraordinary boiling points.

Consumers regularly discover CBD seclude alluring on the grounds that it is without thc. You ought to get that while seclude is adaptable, products dependent on this sort of concentrate are not as compelling as an oil containing a full or wide range cannabinoid profile. The single-cannabinoid profile is less successful because of the absence of cannabinoid and terpene cooperative energies known as the escort effect.Here at Big Sky Botanicals, we produce a wide range product line that contains a full-range profile of cannabinoids and terpenes with just the THC expelled. Since you see how CBD oil is made, make certain to look at how our products are made which layouts the extraction

and preparing strategies we use to make our product line.

CANNABIS PHARMACY OILS AND ITS USAGE

CBD speaks to cannabidiol oil. It is used to treat different appearances notwithstanding the way that its usage is genuinely sketchy. There is moreover some disorder as for how absolutely the oil impacts our bodies. The oil may have medical advantages and such products that have the compound are genuine in various spots today.

Getting THC and CBD

CBD is a cannabinoid, a compound found in cannabis plant. The oil contains CBD centers and the usages change fundamentally. In cannabis, the exacerbate that is remarkable is delta 9 tetrahydrocannabinol or THC. It is a working fixing found in marijuana. Marijuana has CBD and THC and both have different effects.

THC alters the mind when one is smoking or cooking with it. This is in light of the fact that it is isolated by heat. As opposed to THC, CBD is not psychoactive. This infers your point of view doesn't change with use. In any case, critical changes can be noted inside the human body suggesting medical advantages.

Source

Hemp is a bit of the cannabis plant and all around, it isn't dealt with. This is the spot a lot of the CBD is evacuated. Marijuana and hemp start from cannabis sativa, anyway are remarkable. Today, marijuana ranchers are copying plants with the target that they can have high THC levels. Hemp farmers do not need to alter plants and are used to make the CBD oil.

How it Impact the body

Cannabinoids impact the body by interfacing themselves to different receptors. Some cannabinoids are conveyed by the body and there are the CB1 and CB2 receptors. CB1 receptors are discovered all through the body with a dumbfounding number of them being in the cerebrum. The receptors are liable for attitude, emotions, torment, improvement, coordination, memories, craving, thinking, and various limits. THC impacts these receptors.

Concerning the CB2 receptors, they are transcendently in one's protected structure and impact desolation and disturbance. Regardless of the way that CBD does not annex direct here, it manages the body to use cannabinoids more.

The Advantages

CBD is productive to human wellbeing in different ways. It is a trademark distress reliever and has quieting properties. Over the counter medications are used for help with distress and by far most lean toward a dynamically regular other choice and this is the spot CBD oil comes in. Research has shown that CBD gives a predominant treatment, especially for people with relentless torment. There is similarly verification that recommend that the use of CBD can be amazingly helpful for any person who is endeavoring to quit smoking and overseeing drug withdrawals. In an appraisal, it was seen that smokers who had inhalers that had CBD would when all is said in done smoke not as much as what was commonplace for them and with no further needing for cigarettes. CBD could be an unfathomable treatment for people with oppression issue particularly to sedatives.

There are various other medical conditions that are bolstered by CBD and they fuse epilepsy, LGA, Dravet issue, seizures, and so on. More research is being coordinated on the effects of CBD in the human body and the results are empowering. The likelihood of doing combating dangerous development and differing pressure issue is moreover being looked. For all of you who are still on the *Basically Say No* brief prevailing fashion, you may acknowledge that hemp seed oil, which is gotten from the seeds of the cannabis plant, is essentially one more course for those darn radicals to get high. Some time back before administrators and business interests got included, hemp was a noteworthy yield with any advanced and helpful occupations. On the wellbeing front, the seeds of the hemp plant were viewed as a for all intents and purposes immaculate sustenance source, containing 80% of the fundamental unsaturated fats that our bodies need correspondingly as globule edestins which is an unprecedented protein that takes after globulin. Hemp oil is viably consumable and contains for all intents and purposes the aggregate of the central unsaturated fats that the body needs in order to stay working fittingly. Present day Research studies have found that taking hemp oil constantly can help fix a hurt insusceptible structure and even switch wasting making it a critical ordinary upgrade for both sickness patients and people with AIDS.

Taking Internally Cannabis Oil Can:

- Increment essentialness

- Help with engine abilities

- Straightforwardness Arthritis Pain

- Fortify the Immune System

- Treat Tuberculosis

- Reduction Sun Related Damage to the skin

Individuals with conditions brought about by inadequacy in LA (Omega-6) and LNA (Omega-3) can be treated by taking hemp oil since it has those fundamental unsaturated fats (EFA) in adjusted, perfect extents. Hemp seed oil has a low level of Stearic destructive (18:0) which is beneficial for wellbeing since noteworthy degrees of Stearic destructive structure stream blocking clusters in veins and kill the retouching attributes of the EFA's.

The Amount To Take:

On the consistent schedule you can take two-four pastry spoons (up to 50 ml) every day. On account of treatment you can expand the portion up to 150 ml for every day for around seven days, at that point come back to the ordinary day by day sum. Hemp Seed Oil has a nutty flavor that the vast majority find lovely. It is a perfect added substance to plate of mixed greens dressings, plunges, or cold pasta. It is not appropriate for singing, since overabundance warmth will extraordinarily decrease a large number of its nurturing benefits.It can in like manner be used remotely to treat skin conditions, for instance, dermatitis. You can think that its numerous health nourishment stores.

How Hemp Seed Oil Can Help Your Arthritis

There is a colossal issue that exists today with the tremendous number of individuals experiencing joint inflammation in its numerous structures. It is said that well over a large portion of the number of inhabitants in this nation who are more than sixty experience the ill effects of either osteo or rheumatoid joint pain. What the two types of the illness really are I won't go into here, as it is a long and complex subject. Yet, joint pain is a type of irritation which standard medicine seems incapable to address.

Both are brought about by what I call *bone and ligament rock*, the bits of bone and ligament which are left in the joints after the body has begun to decline, focusing on the joints each time it moves. This *rock* rubs on the nerve closes, causing torment, while simultaneously making more harm as the *rock* keeps on scouring endlessly a greater amount of the bone and ligament. As such, an endless loop that modern medicine can not resolve. Be that as it may, there are routes in the elective cure field that may, and I am aware of numerous cases that have, had the option to break this circle.

I suggest that an everyday Hemp Oil Capsule, or the fluid slick, which is very delectable, and can be removed a spoon, ought to be viewed as long haul. Hemp Oil originates from hemp seed:

The Most Nutritionally Complete Food Source In The World.

The Essential Fatty Acids in hemp are renowned for their ability to improve cell advancement and organ limit, Hemp Oil is sensible for Vegetarians and Vegans.

The Use of High-Cannabidiol Cannabis Extracts to Treat Epilepsy and Other Diseases

There has been a passionate climb in news respect for restorative cannabis in 2013, with gives insights about CNN, ABC, CBS, and neighborhood conveyances about high-cannabidiol cannabis oil effectively controlling the indications of unprecedented epileptic conditions like Dravet issue, Doose issue, immature fits, cortical dysplasia, and that is just a hint of something larger. These diseases can make hundreds countless seizures seven days, while moreover blocking headway in different various ways. For families with adolescents encountering such conditions, the troubles are overwhelming. Due to the very astounding nature of Dravet and related issue, standard pharmaceuticals are unable and as often as possible bother the issues. With no other desire, families have gone to high-CBD cannabis oil, which is showing to work with wonderful suitability.

To clarify, high-CBD cannabis oil is non-psychoactive and clearly extensively more critical than high-THC cannabis oil. Cannabidiol is another cannabinoid in the cannabis plant, like the all the all the more striking psychoactive cannabinoid THC, with essential research prescribing neuroprotectant, anticancer, antidiabetic, threatening to ischemic, antispasmodic, antipsychotic, and antibacterial properties, among others. Additionally, cannabis oil is a sort of concentrate from cannabis. Such oil contains a great deal of concentrated cannabinoids that can be orally ingested rather than smoked, securing the therapeutic blends and empowering them to be passed on through stomach related structure, instead of the respiratory system.

The examination prescribes that CBD has panacea-like properties, and before long, this is showing to be the circumstance. On August eleventh, 2013, Sanjay Gupta discharged a record on CNN about Charlotte Figi. Charlotte is a fiery Dravet issue quiet who was having 300 thousand mal seizures seven days. No pharmaceuticals or dietary changes could reasonably diminish this number. Charlotte's kin found a few solutions concerning high-CBD cannabis oil, and after extremely the fundamental piece, Charlotte's seizures halted. She right presently has under three minor seizures a month. This case is completely extraordinary, and it's not isolated. Dr. Margaret Gedde, a Colorado Springs pro, is following eleven new patients of the Stanely family, the suppliers of Charlotte's high-CBD medicine. 9 of them have had 90-100% reduces in seizures, which once more, is essentially superb.

The epileptic conditions that CBD is exhibiting to constrain against are inconceivably amazing, and for no situation the most predominant, all around investigated pharmaceuticals have been prepared for impelling any repairing. Anyway high-CBD cannabis oil is rapidly and seriously reducing reactions, with the fundamental indications being basically useful greater imperativeness, better learning, improved lead, and that is just a hint of something larger.

It should not be astounding that results like these have been proceeding for an extensive period of time. Much equivalent to research shows cannabinoids are remedially feasible against epilepsy, there is research proposing they can crash threatening developments and control distinctive real illnesses. Additionally, before long, for epilepsy and these various conditions, the results are importance individuals. People have been reliably taking out tumors for an extensive period of time and directing contaminations as crohn diabetes, fibromyalgia, coronary disease, consistent torment, various sclerosis, and that is only the start. This is pretty much veritable, more thought must be brought to this issue.essentialness and mental state.

Cannabis Oil a Cancer Treatment Alternative to Chemotherapy?

The THS in cannabis oil connects to the CB2 and CB1 cannabinoid receptors inside of cancerous cells. This leads to an influx of ceramide synthesis, which causes cancer cells to die. The great thing about this is that unlike chemotherapy, cannabis oil only adversely affects cancer cells, not healthy cells. Normal cells do not produce ceramide when exposed to THC, which is why it goes untouched. The cytotoxic chemicals aren't what causes the cancer cells to die - it's the small shift in the mitochondria, which acts as the energy source for cell.

How CBD Oil Helps in Apoptosis

Apoptosis is a characteristic procedure in the body where the cells are decimated as a major aspect of a specific creature's development. As referenced, disease cells develop as an unusual procedure in the body since they never again recognize the body's flag that empower or decimate cell development. As these cells develop and partition, they become increasingly wild. What's more, since they never again react to apoptosis, they will in general speed up cell expansion and disregard different sign from ?typical cells.? That is the reason the endocannabinoid framework is a critical framework in the body since it likewise helps in balancing cell development and demise. As disease cells duplicate quicker than the endocannabinoid framework can deal with, the malignancy cells attack through the typical tissues and spread all through the body. This procedure is called metastasis.

The endocannabinoid framework has two essential receptors. One is the CB1 receptors which are for the most part found in the mind, and the other one is the CB2 receptors which are fundamentally found in the invulnerable framework. THC is the dynamic compound in cannabis that ties to the CB1 receptors and is answerable for state of mind, conduct, and other cerebral capacities. The apoptotic procedure by these receptors is accomplished through the all over again union of ceramide and sphingolipid that advance cell pulverization. When they tie together, the receptor enactment would then be able to help the endocannabinoid framework in flagging an antitumorigenic cautioning. This implies, it impedes malignancy advancement through hindering reproduction, metastasis, and tumor angiogenesis.

With the developing number of states the nation over that have invited enactment making marijuana legitimate, both medically and recreationally, new products are in effect explicitly custom fitted to the maturing populace. One such product, which comes in numerous structures, is Cannabidiol or CBD. CBD which can be conveyed in numerous manners including oil fume, topical cream, ingestible tinctures or edibles, is the non-psychoactive part found in marijuana. In layman terms, CBD conveys the entirety of the advantages of marijuana without making the client high. The constructive outcomes that are expedited utilizing CBD can be especially inviting to seniors.

Numerous seniors don't know about how medical cannabis could improve their personal satisfaction and how the cliché marijuana client and use has changed. Since CBD is extricated from the marijuana plant, seniors can exploit the medical advantages managed by the concentrate without the head or body sensation regularly connected with marijuana. Moreover, seniors have the choice of conveying CBD to their bodies in structures increasingly recognizable, instead of breathing in smoke. CBD is an oil concentrate and consequently can be added to things like topical gels, tinctures and eatable products.

Much of the time, these subordinates of cannabis can lessen or even supplant the utilization of unsafe and addictive professionally prescribed drugs. While this data is just presently advancing into the standard, the characteristic outcome is, seniors drop their preferences, face reality and go to the treatment of their minor and noteworthy age-related diseases using cannabis.

Here are 8 reasons why CBD should turn into a customary piece of each senior's health normal as they age.

1. Help with discomfort

It has for quite some time been realized that cannabis is a torment reliever to a similar degree as, maybe stunningly better, professionally prescribed medicine. For example, clinical investigations have demonstrated that Marijuana is exceptionally successful in diminishing joint pain and nerve torment. Carefully assembled, medical, boutique-style creams are the successful fix of various muscles and joint torments.

2. Bone Health

CBD OilCannabis could give an extraordinary need to the older as it identifies with bone delicacy. As indicated by an examination, cannabis use can help mend cracks and bolster healthier bones. As a result of its calming properties, cannabis can be extremely valuable for patients with different sclerosis.

3. Alleviating Effects

In spite of the fact that CBD is known for its mitigating consequences for senior shoppers, it advances the sentiment of vitality and acts against latency. This is on the grounds that CBD reinforces cells in the human body and adds to finish recovery. What's more, CBD is a cell reinforcement that advances the feeling of carefulness that can be upset by the nearness of free radicals. A study shows that cannabidiol has more grounded cancer prevention agent properties than Vitamin C and Vitamin E.

4. Battles Glaucoma

There has been developing research that supports a connection among cannabis and the treatment of glaucoma. Glaucoma, which is a neurodegenerative malady (the breakdown of neurons in the correspondence procedure from the mind to the body), influences seeing people from an expansion in pressure in the eye known as intraocular pressure (IoP). Returning decades, there is supporting proof that cannabinoids can decrease IoP by up to 25%, anyway the necessary measurement of inward breath of full THC cannabis has represented a hazard to certain patients. Nonetheless, because of the going with manifestations of glaucoma, CBD as a torment the board product functions admirably, and may have the additional advantage of decreasing pressure.

5. A sleeping disorder and Sleep Issues

The more seasoned we get, the more troublesome it is to accomplish continued times of profound rest. During the profound rest stages, our mind recovers and is liberated from poisonous substances, which were delivered by the body itself. Along these lines, rest quality is additionally of colossal significance to avoid age-related neurodegenerative sicknesses, for example, Alzheimer's illness or glaucoma. Every now and again, older individuals are recommended resting pills, which have an incredible potential for reliance and a wide scope of horrendous symptoms. CBD can help in the augmentation of the profound rest stage and the decrease of the lighter dozing stages.

6. Option in contrast to Prescription Medications

The quantity of seniors who utilize every day physician endorsed drugs develops every year pointlessly and persistently. Pharmaceutical organizations present our legislature with one of the biggest campaigning bunches in the nation, to advance the viability and dependability gave by their products. In any case, professionally prescribed drugs can be very perilous for its clients, and can be liable for organ harm, tissue harm, chronic drug use and even demise. In examination, marijuana is a protected option in contrast to physician endorsed drugs, accompanying less symptoms and lower addictive attributes. This advantage is increased with CBD and in reality has been utilized to battle dependence on doctor prescribed drugs. Neither passings nor overdoses have been archived, which are identified with marijuana.

7. Animates Appetite

A general, risky health danger among more established residents is the loss of craving, which causes weight reduction, tissue shortcoming, and mental issues. While marijuana has been widely researched, and appeared to improve the hunger of clients, CBD in like manner has demonstrated to be a decent craving stimulant and along these lines supportive for seniors.

8. Alzheimer's and Dementia

A developing pattern that is being researched is could marijuana forestall the beginning of Alzheimer's illness. As indicated by various investigations, cannabinoids, and by expansion CBD, can add to the end of a dangerous protein identified with this ailment. This is activated by lost aggravation of the mind and recovery of harmed cells.

USEFULNESS OF CANNABIS OIL FOR THE AGED

With the developing number of states the nation over that have invited enactment making marijuana legitimate, both medically and recreationally, new products are as a rule explicitly customized to the maturing populace. One such product, which comes in numerous structures, is Cannabidiol or CBD. CBD which can be conveyed in numerous manners including oil fume, topical cream, ingestible tinctures or edibles, is the non-psychoactive part found in marijuana. In layman terms, CBD conveys the entirety of the advantages of marijuana without making the client high. The beneficial outcomes that are expedited utilizing CBD can be especially inviting to seniors. Numerous seniors don't know about how medical cannabis could improve their personal satisfaction and how the cliché marijuana client and use has changed. Since CBD is removed from the marijuana plant, seniors can exploit the medical advantages managed by the concentrate without the head or body sensation regularly connected with marijuana.

Moreover, seniors have the alternative of conveying CBD to their bodies in structures progressively commonplace, as opposed to breathing in smoke. CBD is an oil concentrate and in this manner can be added to things like topical gels, tinctures and eatable products. Much of the time, these subsidiaries of cannabis can lessen or even supplant the utilization of destructive and addictive professionally prescribed drugs. While this data is just currently advancing into the standard, the characteristic outcome is, seniors drop their partialities, face the truth and go to the treatment of their minor and significant age-related ailments utilizing cannabis.

Here are eight reasons why CBD should turn into a normal part of each senior's health standard as they age.

1. Relief from discomfort

It has for some time been realized that cannabis is a torment reliever to a similar degree as, maybe shockingly better, physician recommended medicine. For example, clinical examinations have demonstrated that Marijuana is exceptionally viable in diminishing joint pain and nerve torment. High quality, medical, boutique-style creams are the powerful fix of various muscles and joint torments.

2. Bone Health

CBD OilCannabis could give an incredible need to the older as it identifies with bone delicacy. As indicated by an examination, cannabis use can help mend breaks and bolster healthier bones. In view of its mitigating properties, cannabis can be exceptionally valuable for patients with various sclerosis.

3. Mitigating Effects

Despite the fact that CBD is known for its relieving consequences for senior purchasers, it advances the sentiment of vitality and acts against latency. This is on the grounds that CBD fortifies cells in the human body and adds to finish recovery. Also, CBD is a cell reinforcement that advances the feeling of carefulness that can be upset by the nearness of free radicals. A study shows that cannabidiol has more grounded cell reinforcement properties than Vitamin C and Vitamin E.

4. Battles Glaucoma

There has been developing research that supports a connection among cannabis and the treatment of glaucoma. Glaucoma, which is a neurodegenerative ailment (the breakdown of neurons in the correspondence procedure from the cerebrum to the body), influences seeing people from an expansion in pressure in the eye known as intraocular pressure (IoP). Returning decades, there is supporting proof that cannabinoids can diminish IoP by up to 25%, anyway the necessary measurement of inward breath of full THC cannabis has represented a hazard to certain patients. Be that as it may, because of the going with side effects of glaucoma, CBD as an agony the executives product functions admirably, and may have the additional advantage of diminishing weight.

5. A Sleeping Disorder And Sleep Issues

The more seasoned we get, the more troublesome it is to accomplish supported times of profound rest. During the profound rest stages, our cerebrum recovers and is liberated from harmful substances, which were delivered by the body itself. Along these lines, rest quality is additionally vital to counteract age-related neurodegenerative sicknesses, for example, Alzheimer's illness or glaucoma. As often as possible, old individuals are recommended dozing pills, which have an extraordinary potential for reliance and a wide scope of upsetting reactions. CBD can help in the expansion of the profound rest stage and the decrease of the lighter dozing stages.

6. Option in contrast to Prescription Medications

The quantity of seniors who utilize every day doctor prescribed drugs develops every year pointlessly and constantly. Pharmaceutical organizations present our legislature with one of the biggest campaigning bunches in the nation, to advance the adequacy and security gave by their products. Be that as it may, doctor prescribed drugs can be incredibly perilous for its clients, and can be liable for organ harm, tissue harm, chronic drug use and even demise. In correlation, marijuana is a protected option in contrast to physician recommended drugs, accompanying less symptoms and lower addictive attributes. This advantage is elevated with CBD and in truth has been utilized to battle dependence on physician endorsed drugs. Neither passings nor overdoses have been recorded, which are identified with marijuana.

7. Animates Appetite

A general, hazardous health danger among more established residents is the loss of craving, which causes weight reduction, tissue shortcoming, and mental issues. While marijuana has been broadly researched, and appeared to improve the hunger of clients, CBD in like manner has demonstrated to be a decent craving stimulant and consequently supportive for seniors.

8. Alzheimer's and Dementia

A rising pattern that is being researched is could marijuana counteract the beginning of Alzheimer's malady. As indicated by various investigations, cannabinoids, and by expansion CBD, can add to the end of a harmful protein identified with this ailment. This is activated by lost irritation of the cerebrum and recovery of damaged cells.

CANNABIS PHARMACY OIL ON PETS

How Is CBD Controlled To Animals?

CBD pet consideration products come in a significant number of similar structures you are most likely used to seeing for people, including edibles (think: chewable treats and cases), oils that can be added to nourishment or set under the tongue and topical creams or emollients that are scoured legitimately on the skin. Like the CBD products implied for people, every one of these CBD pet care product types seems to differently affect the body - in dogs, in any case. When McGrath began examining CBD in 2016, one of her first examinations investigated how three diverse conveyance techniques - a container, an oil and a cream, influenced the way CBD traveled through the assortments of healthy dogs. *"We quantified the pharmacokinetics, which fundamentally implies you give the dogs a solitary portion of every one of the three conveyance strategies and afterward you measure a lot of various blood levels over a 12-hour time frame"* said McGrath. *"So how rapidly is the CBD ingested, how high the blood fixation gets at that solitary portion, and afterward how quick the CBD is killed."*

McGrath found that out of the three explicit plans they tried, the oil had the best pharmacokinetic profile, which means it arrived at the most elevated fixation in the blood, remained in the circulatory system the longest, and played out the most reliably over the various dogs. The case additionally performed well however the cream less so. It performed too conflictingly for McGrath and her group to reach any inferences. These outcomes line up with what we know so far about CBD assimilation in people, yet the research is too primer to be in any way used to settle on any medical choices.

In spite of the fact that there are some topical medications, cannabis oil is regularly managed orally to dogs. It additionally can be utilized related to customary medications and medicines. Rising research proposes there can be *synergistic benefits* among marijuana and conventional medications, Richter sayd: *"There are scarcely any, known critical medication collaborations that you truly should be worried about. Just like the case with any medication, achievement has an inseparable tie to dosing. In the event that you portion pets appropriately, at that point they will get the beneficial outcome that you are searching for while not having any psychoactive symptoms."* But thus lies an issue. The research expected to decide the right measurements for CBD oil in dogs essentially hasn't been done at this point,

Coates says. Also, to exacerbate the situation, FDA testing has indicated that numerous CBD products contain pretty much nothing if any CBD, she includes. The best alternative accessible to pet guardians right now is to converse with a veterinarian who has involvement in pets being treated with cannabis oil about appropriate measurement and trustworthy makers, Coates says.

How does CBD work in animals?

It is hazy, and a riddle researchers are as yet attempting to unravel in people too. For example, dogs have an endocannabinoid framework however whether CBD communicates with it similarly specialists figure it does in people is not yet clear. For the present, all McGrath knows is that in dogs, as in people, CBD seems, by all accounts, to be utilized by the liver.

Are there any health advantages to giving your pet CBD?

Once more, it is too soon to tell. A recent report found that CBD can assist increment with encouraging and action in dogs with osteoarthritis and the next year McGrath distributed an examination demonstrating CBD may help lessen the quantity of seizures experienced by epileptic dogs. In any case, despite the fact that these examinations were well-planned and peer-evaluated, they're still little and extremely starter. *"All we have essentially done is give this medication to these dogs and stated, OK, this is what we're seeing"* says McGrath. *"Yet, regardless of whether the blood levels accomplished are sufficient enough to treat certain ailments, we do not yet have the foggiest idea".* Veterinarians do not have a wide assortment of drugs accessible to treat these conditions and a portion of the ones that do exist regularly accompany weakening reactions, for example, weight increase and laziness. *"On the off chance that CBD works, at that point I figure it would hit the sign of being both successful and not conveying a ton of symptoms. So, sort of what we are seeking after."* said McGrath

McGrath and different researchers across the country are at present leading bigger investigations on CBD's adequacy in treating osteoarthritis in dogs and cats, epilepsy in dogs and post-employable torment, yet it will be some time before the outcomes are distributed. Until more is known, it is ideal to converse with your veterinarian before giving your creature CBD.

Is CBD safe for animals?

CBD, in its unadulterated state, radiates an impression of being ensured and well-suffered by animals, as showed by a 2017 World Health Organization report. Regardless, both resulting 2018 canine examinations referenced above saw an extension in the liver substance solvent phosphatase (ALP) during CBD treatment. As a segment of her assessment, McGrath ran a simultaneous liver limit test to guarantee the dogs' livers were not missing the mark and everything returned commonplace so it is dim whether the raised ALP levels were achieved by something absolutely positive or could shape into a continuously significant issue whole deal. *"I would be a little stressed over offering CBD to a canine that has known liver issues"* says McGrath. Furthermore, because CBD has every one of the reserves of being prepared by the liver, McGrath says she would similarly be careful about offering CBD to a canine who starting at now takes a solution that is used by the liver. *"We don't by and large have the foggiest thought regarding these things interface right now"* she says. The different colossal thing pet owners should think about is quality control. Since the CBD market is not especially overseen now, CBD products can contain fixings that are not recorded on their names, including THC, which is known to be hazardous to cats and dogs.

One way to deal with avoid perhaps hazardous fixings is to simply use products that go with a confirmation of assessment, or COA (the cluster number on the COA should arrange the number on the product's name or packaging). A COA is given when a self-sufficient lab tests the product to assert its fixings and quality, notwithstanding different things. Genuinely, CBD products must contain near 0.3% THC, which should be okay for animals. Nonetheless, there's no inspiration to go for broke. At whatever point possible, stick to CBD pet thought products that contain 0.0% THC and be attentive for signs of THC hurting, for instance, spewing, detachment of the entrails, torpidity, tension and issue standing. Essential concern: *"We haven't found whatever's excessively upsetting about CBD. However, on the opposite side, in spite of all that we know beside no about it and it's very critical for owners to understand that and use it with alert until we have more information"* says McGrath.

What Are the Benefits of Cannabis Oil for Dogs?

Cannabis oil can be used to treat seizures, ailment, stress, pressure, joint aggravation, back desolation, appearances of dangerous development, and gastrointestinal issues, among other wellbeing conditions in dogs. Help is given as the cannabinoids in marijuana work together with the endocannabinoid system, Shu explains. *"It's a movement of receptors that run all through the body. The cannabinoids team up with the receptors in the body and direct things like torment, uneasiness, and nausea."* Unlike some ordinary torment medicine for dogs, medical cannabis has no unsafe responses with authentic portion, Shu points out: *"It does not hurt the kidney, liver, or GI tract. The dogs are not high or quieted."*

What Are the Potential Risks of Cannabis Oil for Pets?

Like any meds, overdosing can incite potential dangers for pets. *"The most huge is THC dangerous quality, which infers, basically, they are high. Subordinate upon how unmitigated a pet has been overdosed, the impacts of that can be amazingly enduring, even days"* said Richter. During these scenes, a pet will no doubt be not capable stand or eat. On the off chance that you accept an overdose, take your pet to the veterinarian right away. Dangerous dangers for dogs from medical cannabis are *exceedingly striking*, Richter says, including that lethality much more periodically happens when a pet has eaten a product that contains chocolate, espresso, or raisins. *"In spite of whether the THC harmful quality is not outrageous, they can a segment of the time have issues because of these different fixings."* That communicated, ingestion of a huge amount of marijuana has been fatal in various dogs, so defeating overdoses with medical cannabis is so far fundamental, cautions Dr. Jennifer Coates, a veterinary expert with petMD.

Graham Quigley, proprietor and acupuncturist at the Holistic Animal Clinic in San Rafael, California, centers around that as the normality of elective medicine amasses, pet guards may get tied up with *irrationally aching cases about cannabis oil* from defective sources. Quigley stresses that cannabis oil is not a *fix all*. As with any medicine, pet guards should coordinate their veterinarian first before treating their canine with cannabis oil.

Where Can Pet Owners Get Cannabis Oil for Their Dogs?

Getting medical cannabis for your pet all depends upon where you live and your state's marijuana laws. *"In California, to legitimately buy marijuana, you should have a medical cannabis card, which an individual would get from their primary care physician. There is no lawful system by which I, as a veterinarian, can give a medical cannabis card to a pet"* Richter says. Pet owners who need to give their pooch cannabis oil should address their veterinarian. From that point, pet guardians who have a medical marijuana card can visit a legitimate dispensary and buy the product that best addresses their pet's issues. Pet guardians who live in areas where medical marijuana isn't accessible can likewise think about hemp products, which have lower portions of THC.

NEGATIVE IMPLICATIONS OF CANNABIS ABUSE ON GENERAL AND ORAL HEALTH

Cannabis, normally known as Marijuana, is the most as often as possible utilized unlawful medication in America. As indicated by National Survey on Drug Use and Health (NSDUH), there were about 15.2 million past month clients in America in 2008. It additionally expressed that about 2.2 million individuals utilized Marijuana without precedent for 2008.

This midpoints to around sixthousand Marijuana starts for each day. Numerous individuals are getting dependent on Marijuana, unmindful of its destructive consequences for health. Today, Cannabis abuse is a huge worry because of its negative effects on general physical, mental and oral wellbeing.

There are three principle types of Cannabis: Marijuana, Hash and Hash oil, all of which contain the fundamental psychoactive constituent, Delta-9-Tetrahydrocannabinol, just called as THC. Cannabis misuse influences pretty much every arrangement of the body including the cardiovascular, respiratory, mental and oral frameworks.

A portion of the negative ramifications of Cannabis misuse are:

Impacts on general health

At the point when somebody smokes or devours Cannabis, THC goes from the lungs or stomach into the circulation system, which conveys the substance to the cerebrum and different organs all through the body. As indicated by National Institute on Drug Abuse (NIDA), pulse is expanded by twenty to hundred percent not long after smoking Marijuana.

It is additionally evaluated that Marijuana clients have very nearly multiple times danger of coronary episode in the principal hour in the wake of smoking Marijuana. Maturing individuals or those with heart vulnerabilities will be at higher hazard. Long haul smoking of Marijuana is related with negative impacts on the respiratory framework. The smoke from a Cannabis cigarette has indistinguishable substance from tobacco smoke separated from unsafe substance like carbon monoxide, bronchial aggravations, tar and more significant levels of different cancer-causing agents than in tobacco smoke. Constant smokers of Cannabis have expanded side effects of bronchitis, including hacking, wheezing, mucus production, increasingly visit intense chest ailment, and expanded danger of lung diseases.

The manifestations of bronchitis are more typical in Cannabis smokers than non-smokers of the medication. Cannabis misuse results in dysregulated development of epithelial cells in lungs, which may prompt malignancy.

Consequences for mental health

Intense impacts of Cannabis misuse fluctuate extraordinarily between people contingent upon the measurements, technique for organization, condition and character of the client. Long haul Cannabis misuse expands the danger of genuine mental diseases. THC follows up on explicit locales in the mind, called cannabinoid receptors. The most noteworthy thickness of cannabinoid receptors are found in parts of the cerebrum that impact joy, memory, musings, focus, tangible and time discernment and so forth. Clearly, Marijuana inebriation can cause misshaped recognitions, debilitated coordination, trouble in intuition and critical thinking, and issues with learning and memory. Marijuana misuse can expand paces of uneasiness, despondency, self-destructive ideation, and schizophrenia.

Effects on oral health

Cannabis clients are inclined to oral diseases. By and large, Cannabis abusers have more unfortunate oral health than non-clients, with higher rotted, absent and filled (DMF) teeth scores, higher plaque scores and less healthy teeth gums. A significant reaction of Cannabis misuse is xerostomia (dryness of the mouth brought about by failing salivary organs). Cannabis smoking and biting causes changes in the oral epithelium, named *cannabis stomatitis*. Its side effects incorporate aggravation and shallow anesthesia of the oral membranous tissue covering inner organs. With ceaseless use, this may advance to neoplasia (development of a tumor).

Cannabis use causes oral malignant growth

Constant smokers of Cannabis have an expanded danger of creating oral leukoplakia (thick white fixes on mucous films of the oral cavity, including the tongue. It frequently happens as a pre-malignant development), oral disease and other oral contaminations. Oral malignancy identified with cannabis as a rule happens on the foremost floor of the mouth and the tongue. Cannabis utilization additionally has its effects on driving, influencing engine abilities, reflexes, and consideration. This builds coincidental dangers. Cannabis misuse can possibly mess up day by day life too. Cannabis misuse disables a few significant proportions of life accomplishment including physical and mental health, psychological capacities, public activity and profession status. The expanding commonness of Cannabis use requests familiarity with the different unfavorable effects of Cannabis misuse. Individuals should think about these effects and make auspicious move so as to avoid its negative ramifications.

RELATED EFFECTS ON USAGE OF CANNABIS PHARMACY OIL

Late studies have uncovered many of its advantages and introduced proof of its potential as an a lot more secure alternative over numerous pharmaceutical drugs. Notwithstanding, there is still a great deal to be wanted as far research on this non-psychoactive cannabinoid is concerned. Because of the absence of broad investigation on its symptoms, it is frequently not exhorted by specialists even in places where medical marijuana is legitimate. Despite its advantages, this home grown concentrate, such as everything else we can ingest or use on ourselves, has certain symptoms. To comprehend the suitability of this medication as a potential solution for various illnesses, it is basic for us to think about CBD oil's reactions in some detail.

Unexpectedly, no instances of danger or overdose from utilization of hemp-based (modern evaluation hemp) CBD oil have been accounted for up until now. Actually, this specific concentrate of marijuana or hemp has been seen as very safe for use by nearly everybody. Dosages of up to 1500mg of CBD have been believed to be effectively endured by human. Portions of up to 1500mg of CBD have been believed to be effectively endured by human guineas pigs. CBD scarcely has any negative effect on people, may happen just in uncommon cases and that too in a gentle manner.

Be that as it may, there are connected effects on the use of CBD oil which are examined underneath;

- **Mouth Dryness:** This is a typical wonder among individuals who use CBD or some other cannabinoids, in the two instances of expending or smoking. A wonder, which feels like your mouth is loaded down with cotton balls, can be effectively overwhelmed by drinking a great deal of water or other hydrating liquids previously, during or after utilization of CBD. The explanation behind this is the point at which an individual devours or smokes any cannabinoid, the endocannabinoid framework, which has its receptors present in the salivary organs, represses the discharge of the organs. Ongoing considers (one) have found that the submandibular organ that produces over 60% of the spit has cannabinoid receptors. Anandamide,an endocannabinoid that causes dryness of mouth, interfaces with these receptors and hinders salivation production by obstructing the sign from the sensory system to create spit.

- **Sluggishness:** CBD oil regularly does not incite any sentiments of languor. Be that as it may, CBD's impact on people varies from individual to individual. As a rule, CBD has a wake-inciting impact, making an individual progressively alert and enthusiastic, while in others it can create the exact inverse response. In extremely high portions, the last classification of individuals has detailed inclination lazy in the wake of expending CBD. Diminishing the measurement can be a decent alternative. On the off chance that you have a place with this class of individuals, it is best for you to NOT work any substantial hardware or drive a vehicle, for your very own wellbeing and people around you. As another safety measure for individuals who experience sluggishness because of devouring CBD oil, lessening the dose can be a decent alternative.

- **Dazedness or Lightheadedness**: some tea or espresso can do some amazing things in such circumstances. A truly uncommon and impermanent reaction, unsteadiness can be effectively overseen by drinking a stimulated refreshment that will help your body rapidly recapture its typical equalization. Some tea or espresso can do some amazing things in such circumstances, yet try to drink a great deal of water alongside it, as caffeine has a drying out impact on the body.

- **Drop in Blood Pressure**: This is normally the motivation behind why a few people experience wooziness. While there is proof of CBD oil helping individuals with heart sicknesses and diabetes by bringing down their pulse, this nature of this cannabinoid can have negative effect on individuals with ordinary circulatory strain. As indicated by certain investigations, higher portions of CBD can cause a slight drop in pulse. Any product containing over 0.3% THC is Illegal. Along these lines, individuals who experience the ill effects of low circulatory strain or are taking medicine for it should cease from devouring CBD or CBD-based products. While it is in every case best to counsel a specialist before considering CBD oil as an elective treatment, whenever looked with such a circumstance, drinking espresso typically helps, much the same as if there should be an occurrence of wooziness.

- **Diarrhea and Change in Appetite and Weight:** In 2017, a clinical investigation of patients with epilepsy and insane issue and their response to CBD oil as a type of treatment was distributed in the diary, Cannabis and Cannabinoid Research. Over the span of their research, researchers found that the subjects encountered some regular symptoms like tiredness, loose bowels, and changes in both weight as well as hunger. Be that as it may, it was reasoned that: *"In examination with different drugs, utilized for the treatment of these medical conditions, CBD has a superior reaction profile."* This study, in any case, left space for progressively broad research into the *toxicological parameters* of CBD oil, for occasion, its impact on hormones.

- **Impact on Patients with Movement Disorders**: A couple of increasingly potential threats of CBD use do even now exist, especially among patients of some prior conditions, for instance, among patients of dystonic development issue. Patients when treated with oral dosages of 100–600mg CBD oil every day. In an investigation, distributed in the International Journal of Neuroscience in 2009, such patients when treated with oral portions of 100–600mg CBD oil every day for a time of about a month and a half, close by standard prescriptions, gave indications of progress. In any case, that was likewise joined by the regular symptoms referenced above (low circulatory strain, dryness of mouth, languor and wooziness), alongside not really basic psychomotor easing back (or backing off of point of view and of physical developments). At the point when the portion was over 300 mg/day,symptoms like increment in hypokinesia and resting tremor were seen, uncovering one of the threats of utilizing CBD oil on patients of Parkinson's Disease. However, another examination , distributed in the Journal of Psychopharmacology recommended that utilization of CBD really improves the personal satisfaction in patients with Parkinson's disease.This goes to demonstrate that a great deal of research should be done around there to determine at an authoritative end in regards to the advantage as well as negative effect on patients of Parkinson's Disease.

Interaction with Pharmaceutical Drugs

Individuals taking any pharmaceutical prescription for a previous affliction or condition must be especially cautious about CBD's effects on medicate digestion inside the liver. CBD has been found to obstruct the movement of specific chemicals found in the liver, for example, the cytochrome P450 compound framework (especially CYP3A4) – that processes pharmaceutical drugs implied for human utilization. P450 chemical framework contains in excess of fifty compounds. As indicated by Davis' Drug Guide, the P450 chemical framework contains in excess of fifty proteins that procedure and dispose of poisons. (seven) If taken in high dosages, CBD oil can totally kill P450 protein's movement, as this cannabinoid requires a similar chemical to be processed. In addition, certain pharmaceutical drugs additionally restrain this protein. This mean the breakdown of CBD oil may get upset prompting an expansion in its physiological action. Besides, there are sure pharmaceutical prescriptions that can really expand the degree of this chemical, bringing about quicker breakdown of CBD. Albeit such impedances may just be a minor and generally a brief issue, it is constantly protected to counsel your primary care physician before utilizing CBD oil alongside pharmaceutical drugs.

Reactions of FDA-Approved Drug for Epilepsy

The US Food and Drug Administration endorsed Epidiolex (a CBD-based medication) oral answer for treatment of two kinds of epilepsy , Lennox-Gastaut Syndrome and Dravet Syndrome for patients matured 2 years or more. Be that as it may, throughout its clinical preliminaries, researchers found certain unfavorable effects (6) of the medication:

- Liver issues

- Manifestations identified with the focal sensory system like peevishness and torpidity

- Diminished hunger

- Gastrointestinal issues

- Diseases

- Rashes and other affectability responses

- Diminished pee

- Breathing issues

- Danger of intensifying emotional episodes, wretchedness or self-destructive propensities.

What Are the Drugs That Cbd Interacts With?

CBD (as talked about prior) restrains the breakdown of certain pharmaceutical drugs and, now and again, the other way around. This may prompt the nearness of more significant levels of these drugs in your framework, causing undesirable symptoms, now and then even an overdose. It is basic to take note of that CBD oil isn't the only one in this impact on medicate digestion. Grapefruit, watercress, St John's Wort, and goldenseal likewise hinder movement of the cytochrome P450 or CYP450.The drugs being referred to, any medication that requires the liver's CYP450 chemicals to utilize might associate with CBD oil. As indicated by the Indiana

University Department of Medicine, drugs known to utilize the CYP450 framework incorporate (seven):

- Steroids

- HMG CoA reductase inhibitors

- Calcium channel blockers

- Antihistamines

- Prokinetics

- HIV antivirals

- Insusceptible modulators

- Benzodiazepines

- Antiarrythmics

- Anti-infection agents

- Sedatives

- Antipsychotics

- Antidepressants

- Enemies of epileptics

- Beta blockers

- PPIs

- NSAIDs

- Angiotension II blockers

- Oral hypoglycemic specialists

- Sulfonylureas

It must be referenced here that this rundown is not thorough and neither would it be able to be said with vindication that every one of these drugs will unfavorably respond with cannabidiol. It is best for you to counsel a medical expert before enhancing your treatment with CBD oil.

Prodrug

There is additionally a gathering of medicines that fall under the *prodrug* classification. These are meds that should be used to the restorative compound. In other words, when you ingest an inert compound, it enters your framework and is then prepared into a functioning medication. In the event that this handling requires CYP3A4 (some portion of the bigger CYP450 framework), at that point CBD can hinder the response, leaving too minimal dynamic medication in the body for the ideal effect. Case in point: Codeine that is processed into morphine. Vyvanse and Concerta are two other pharmaceutical meds, implied for ADHD, which likewise fall under this classification.

Wellbeing Concerns

Cannabis is getting very well known as a protected and characteristic medicine, with for all intents and purposes zero lethality. Research has appraised this cannabinoid as least hazardous substance, when contrasted with substances, for example, liquor and nicotine concerning toxicity. But the inquiry is: Is CBD a characteristic nourishment supplement or a medicine? Most talks identifying with its lawful status relies upon that, since "restorative drugs are viewed as risky until demonstrated safe" while it is the polar opposite if there should arise an occurrence of characteristic supplements.

Additionally, CBD oil is as yet unregulated, which means its right measurement is as yet obscure. Be that as it may, human examinations have demonstrated that CBD is very all around endured even up to a day by day portion of 1,500mg. Cannabidiol is nearly sheltered when expended in proper dosages among grown-ups. CBD portions of up to 300mg day by day have been utilized securely for as long as a half year. ortions of 1200-1500mg day by day have been utilized securely for as long as about a month. Cannabidiol under-the-tongue showers have been utilized in portions of 2.5mg for as long as about fourteen days.

Believe it or not, as demonstrated by a progressing World Health Organization (WHO) review: *"until this point in time, there is no evidence of recreational use of CBD or any broad wellbeing related issues related with the use of unadulterated CBD"*. While the unadulterated type of CBD might be of a lot of advantage to mankind, the fundamental concern is the sythesis of the products that are being made accessible in the market. Here, we are discussing the nearness of Tetrahydrocannabinol (or THC) (instances of mislabeling) and contaminants.

Mislabeling: According to research paper distributed in the Journal of the American Medical Association in 2017, practically 70% of all CBD products sold online are mislabeled. This implies they could contain higher hints of THC (just 0.3% and lower is allowed in modern evaluation CBD or hemp oil) that could genuinely hurt patients with tension issue and other maniacal issue. Contaminants: Studies have uncovered that cannabis plants from uncontrolled sources might be polluted with different destructive substances that could prompt serious health risks. Contaminants that are for the most part included by makers incorporate synthetic concoctions added purposefully to increase its yield, weight, or power:

- Pesticides

- Metal particles

- Engineered cannabinoids (Fake pot) (fifteen)

- Certain different components that may enter the plant accidentally are:

- Overwhelming metals

- Molds and microscopic organisms

- Aflatoxins

A valid example: An ongoing paper from the Netherlands Ministry of Environment and Health uncovered that more than 90% of the Dutch cannabis sold in cafés contains hints of unlawful yield security Items such as pesticides.

(16) Another case: pesticides are also found in cannabis sold under state law in California

[17] as well as in regenerative cannabis from licensed producers in Canada.

[18].The uplifting news is that most contaminants are very simple to recognize, on account of the presence of the numerous expert logical labs that routinely screen for such contaminants in nourishment crops, imported

therapeutic plants or eatable oils. Similar lab techniques can be applied to test for contaminants in CBD oils.

When Should You Avoid CBD Oil?

While CBD oil has numerous restorative effects on the human body and psyche, there are times and circumstances when you ought to avoid CBD oil utilization or use.

During Pregnancy

There is proof of the sick effects of marijuana products on babies, if the mother is utilizing it during her pregnancy or while she is as yet breastfeeding her youngster (twenty, twenty-one and twenty-two). Be that as it may, there is no such proof with respect to CBD in its unaltered structure, which has only 0.3 per cent THC and no more. As indicated by certain researchers, since cannabinoid receptors are engaged with mental health, CBD oil may upset fetal mental health. In any case, others are of the sentiment that CBD may, truth be told, advance healthy fetal mental health, since CBD can advance neurogenesis.

Awful for Children beneath two Years of Age

Without legitimate guidelines and adequate watchfulness over the closeout of CBD products, it isn't protected to oversee CBD in any structure to infants and kids underneath the age of two years. What impact even the small hints of THC may have on your infant and whether your child may get influenced by the following components of contaminants are not dangers you would need to take with your little one's health. It is ideal to guarantee you are utilizing CBD in its most perfect structure and that too simply in the wake of counseling a specialist experienced in CBD's effects.

When Taking Antipsychotic, Antidepressant Drugs

This has been clarified before in *what are the drugs that CBD connects with?* and a sub-segment *under are there any reactions to utilizing CBD oil?*

Outline

Despite its security concerns, it is verifiable how many individuals are progressively picking CBD products over pharmaceutical ones for the treatment of various illnesses, both physical and mental. This is generally because of its fewer reactions and by nil possibility of overdosing. Exploiting the ascent popular, a lot of corrupt makers and cannabis cultivators have come into the business with the sole expectation of profiting, without paying a lot of thought to the welfare of the individuals to whom they sell their products. In line with this, it is up to us as buyers to be careful and to do our own research before we take the risk of CBD products accessible on the market, in particular online ones.

Before getting into the particular advantages of cannabis oil, it's critical to comprehend the various kinds of cannabis oil that are available.Cannabis and hemp plants contain diverse cannabinoids. These are substance parts that have some impact on you when expended. The two most regular cannabinoids are THC and CBD. Many tinctures, oils and cannabis products currently contain a certain proportion of THC and CBD. THC is the one that has brought the *high* to the vast majority of marijuana partners. Once, CBD is commonly used for restorative purposes.

The principle sorts of cannabis oil include:

CBD oil. This is a nonpsychoactive cannabis product. It doesn't contain THC, so it won't deliver a *high*. CBD oil is prized for its restorative effects, including facilitating uneasiness, agony, and symptoms of chemotherapy.

Hemp-determined oil. Hemp is fundamentally the same as the cannabis plant, however it does not have any THC. It can contain CBD, yet its quality is typically viewed as the second rate. All things considered, hemp-determined oil can be a decent choice on the off chance that you live in a territory that has not legitimized cannabis.

Marijuana-inferred oil. Cannabis oil separated from a similar plant as dried marijuana leaves and buds has a higher proportion of THC. Subsequently, it has psychoactive effects.

Rick Simpson Oil (Rso). RSO contains elevated levels of THC with next to zero CBD. When picking a cannabis oil, make a point to deliberately take a gander at the name so you comprehend what proportion of THC to CBD you are getting.

Hemp Oil versus CBD Oil

Most strikingly, the various terms to portray hemp, CBD and the different hemp-inferred products are particularly confounding. Huge numbers of the words are utilized reciprocally, however can mean altogether different things.

Is it hemp oil? CBD oil? Hemp seed oil? Shouldn't something is said about Hemp CBD to extricate? At that point there is cannabis oil, marijuana remove, the rundown continues forever.

Numerous enormous purchaser brands are likewise hopping onto the CBD temporary fad from CVS to Ben and Jerry's Ice Cream to Coca Cola. While these are unquestionably energizing occasions for the business, it's critical to comprehend the wording and truly realize what you're obtaining. The expression *hemp oil* may allude to either hemp seed oil or CBD oil, however CBD oil ought to never be utilized to portray hemp seed oil, I know, confounding!

While both hemp seed oil and CBD oil share certain attributes, and both have their advantages, there are some significant contrasts. In this book, we will concentrate on the contrasts between hemp seed oil and CBD Oil.

So, first of all, how do we characterize a few terms:

Cannabis:

Cannabis is a plant in the family Cannabaceae, beginning from Central Asia. There are three fundamental types of cannabis:

- Cannabis Indica

- Cannabis Sativa

- Cannabis Ruderalis

Marijuana

Marijuana is an assortment of cannabis sativa that contains a high measure of THC, which is the concoction (cannabinoid) liable for its inebriating effects. Marijuana is utilized for both medical or potentially recreational purposes. On account of marijuana's high THC content and psychoactive properties, it has been esteemed unlawful in numerous pieces of the world, including the US. Despite the fact that an ever increasing number of states are sanctioning recreational marijuana as of late, it stays delegated a Schedule 1 medication on a government level.

Hemp

Like marijuana, hemp is another assortment of cannabis sativa, however has a much lower convergence of THC (0.3% or less). Hemp is broadly collected for modern uses, for example, paper, development materials and materials. In light of the low measure of THC, hemp has likewise been developed for non-tranquilize use as a health supplement.

CBD

CBD represents Cannabidiol. CBD is a concoction compound found in cannabis and has numerous therapeutic advantages, for example, calming and hostile to nervousness properties with no psychoactive effects.

CBD is available in all cannabis strains, including both marijuana and hemp assortments.

Note: CBD got from marijuana is as yet illicit in the US because of the high THC content in marijauana. Hemp-determined CBD is governmentally legitimate in the US under the 2018 Farm Bill since hemp contains under 0.3% THC. In this way, the lawfulness of CBD lies in the key expression "got from hemp".

What Is Hemp Seed Oil?

Hemp seed oil, which is here and there alluded to as hemp oil, is extricated by cool squeezing the seeds of the hemp plant. This is like how olive oil or coconut oil is sourced. The hemp seed oil has been accessible in health nourishment stores for quite a long time. It very well may be found in products, for example, cooking oil, moisturizers, skin care, beauty care products and cleansers.

What's the value of Hemp Seed Oil?

Hemp seed oil is known as a superfood because it contains high levels of cancer prevention agents, vitamins, minerals and amino acids. Hemp seeds contain huge measures of omega-3 and omega-6 unsaturated fats, which can help decrease the indications of maturing, improve cardiovascular health and add to bring down the cholesterol levels. Hemp seeds are an extraordinary plant based wellspring of protein, which makes hemp seed oil an ideal wellspring of complete protein for veggie lovers and vegetarians. Hemp seed oil is additionally an incredible lotion, and can be utilized to help hydrate your hair, nails and skin without stopping up your pores.

As a result of hemp seed's numerous health and nourishing advantages, everybody could utilize somewhat more hemp seed oil in their lives. The main downside of the hemp seed oil is that it does not contain any cannabinoids (THC, CBD, and so on), terpenes or other therapeutic mixes found in the stalks, leaves and blooms of the cannabis plant. This implies it does not furnish any of the advantages related to entire plant hemp separates.

What is CBD Oil?

CBD oil is gotten from the stalks, leaves and blooms (*airborne parts*) of the cannabis plant. Since the hemp strain of cannabis contains low degrees of THC, CBD got from hemp won't make you *high*. The proportion of high

CBD to low THC makes hemp plants perfect for making CBD oil (and lawful!). CBD oil is removed from hemp utilizing either ethanol or CO_2 extraction process more on that later. There are various kinds of CBD oil extricated from hemp including full range, expansive range and CBD confine. For a point by point clarification about the upsides and downsides of each, read our past post here. CBD oil can once in a while be alluded to as CBD extricate, hemp removes or phytocannabinoid-rich (PCR) hemp separate.

What are the Benefits of CBD oil?

CBD oil got from hemp works with the body through the endocannabinoid framework (ECS). The endocannabinoid framework is liable for advancing homeostasis, which is the body's capacity to keep up parity and capacity appropriately. The ECS is ensnared is managing a significant number of our body's capacities, for example, rest, state of mind, torment, craving, hormone, and resistant reaction.

Taking CBD oil can help with an assortment of health related issues, for example,

- Nervousness and sadness

- Relief from discomfort

- Hostile to aggravation

- Rest conditions

- Neurological issue

- Substance misuse

- Intellectual capacities

- Significance of Knowing the Difference

Run a quest on Amazon for CBD oil and you'll discover plenty of *Hemp Oil* products, yet what does that really mean? Clue: it is presumably not what you think. In the event that you unwittingly buy hemp seed oil thinking you'll receive the rewards of CBD, you will be significantly frustrated. Likewise, removing CBD oil is a substantially more muddled procedure than cold squeezing hemp seeds, along these lines CBD oil products are significantly more costly contrasted with hemp seed oil. A few advertisers are attempting to get on board with the CBD temporary fad and advancing hemp seed oil in a similar way as CBD, fooling purchasers into paying a premium for regular hemp seed oil. On the off chance that you fall prey to this strategy, your wallet will likewise be enormously frustrated. It is likewise critical to comprehend what to search for when purchasing CBD products. Unfortunately, most companies falsely say that their drug gives CBD, when it does not contain any.

What to Look For When You Buy CBD Oil

Hemp seed oil is generally straight forward as far as naming is concerned. It's an alternative story for CBD products. Using your new phrase learning will significantly allow you to decode what you need to look for when assessing CBD oil products. If you're interested in trying CBD just because, start by reading our Beginner's CBD Guide. *Here are some extra tips:*

1. Ensure you read the marks to guarantee that CBD, Cannabidiol or *Phytocannabinoid-rich (PCR) hemp* is recorded as fixing just as the sum recorded, regularly in milligrams.

2. Ensure you know whether the product contains any THC. A few people will most likely be unable to ingest THC because of lawful purposes, breezing through a medication test, or some other individual reasons.

3. Ask what extraction strategy is utilized to remove CBD from hemp. Indication: CO_2 extraction is free of unsafe solvents and utilizations a delicate, low temperature, liquor free extraction process that yields the most flawless type of CBD Oil.

4. Read through COA's (Certificate of Analysis) and lab test results to guarantee they can back up their cases.

5. Find out about the organization, its notoriety and their arrival approach. Ensure they can address any inquiries or concerns you have about their products.

6. Peruse online audits for the products you are considering to check whether others have encountered positive outcomes.

Key Takeaways

- Marijuana and hemp are two unique strains of the cannabis plant.

- Hemp seed oil originates from hemp, while CBD oil can be obtained from either marijuana or hemp.

- Hemp seed oil and CBD oil have both their advantages, although there are significant differences between them.Hemp seed oil is separated by chilly squeezing hemp seeds, while CBD oil is extricated from the stalks, leaves and blooms of the plant.

- *Hemp oil* may allude to either hemp seed oil or CBD oil.

ALTERNATIVES TO CANNABIS PHARMACY OIL

Medication testing has gotten normal in numerous working environments, and obligatory for those in government positions, law authorization, avionics, health and crisis medical consideration, and sports (especially those tried for prohibited substances). What numerous CBD clients do not understand is that follow measures of THC (the psychoactive compound in cannabis) can be found in CBD products, representing a potential danger of a positive medication test. All in all, what do you do in case you're medication tried in your calling, yet need to encounter the health advantages of CBD? You can either avoid the substance through and through or you can take a safe CBD elective that takes a shot at your endocannabinoid framework superior to CBD alone.

How the Endocannabinoid System Works

To start with, it is critical to comprehend the endocannabinoid framework or ECS. You might be acquainted with this generally new term yet at the same time confounded about what it is actually. The endocannabinoid framework is six-hundred-million-years of age, yet as of late found in the late '80s by a researcher researching the cannabis plant. What researchers found was a complex and wise body-wide receptor site framework that is responsible for managing rest wake cycles, temperament, tension and stress, digestion, vitality, agony and irritation, mental health, and much more.

While it has nothing to do with getting *high*, the ECS is an unbelievably significant framework that has a vital influence in the guideline, upkeep, and parity of ideal health and recuperating. *"The ECS with its activities in our resistant framework, sensory system, and all the body's organs, is truly a scaffold among body and brain"* says Dustin Sulak.

How CBD Affects the Body

Since you discover somewhat more about how the ECS functions, we should plunge into how CBD collaborates with this framework and influences the body. Your endocannabinoid framework requires *activators* called cannabinoids. Some cannabinoids are created normally in your body, called endocannabinoids and others are gotten from plants (like hemp or cannabis) called phytocannabinoids. These cannabinoids tie to receptor locales (CB1 and CB2) like a key does to a lock and may discharge a perplexing course of synapses that impart essential data to cells, tissues, organs, and organs basic to keeping up ideal health and homeostasis. In any case, researchers have found many non-cannabis and non-hemp plants that additionally contain mending phytocannabinoids that can initiate and support the endocannabinoid framework. This implies you can accomplish similar outcomes with different alternatives.

Did you say Non-Cannabis Cannabinoids?

Truly, believe it or not. Furthermore, you may as of now be acquainted with a portion of these non-cannabis plants, for example, ginger, echinacea and clove oil. Non-cannabis plants can imitate the movement of cannabinoids yet have an alternate structure called cannabimimetic mixes and might be more successful at enacting the endocannabinoid framework than CBD alone. This is particularly incredible news for people who can not take CBD or who need to avoid the shame of cannabis and hemp.

All in all, what are the names of these non-cannabis cannabinoids?

Here is a short rundown of probably the most dominant herbs and botanicals containing phytocannabinoids that can assume a key job in your health.

Ginger root: One of the most powerful mitigating plants, ginger root is wealthy in the two cell reinforcements and cannabinoids. Since irritation can significantly affect your tissues, muscles, and joints, ginger root is basic to incorporate into your eating regimen. It normally supports the ECS by connecting to receptors liable for managing agony and aggravation.

- **Magnolia:** Experts have found that magnolia bark and its fundamental bioactive mixes (magnolol and honokiol) have calming, hostile to bacterial and against unfavorably susceptible specialists. Moreover, magnolia can initiate cannabinoid receptors answerable for controlling rest, memory, and uneasiness.

- **Dark pepper:** This powerful herb ties with CB2 receptors liable for directing irritation and torment. In view of its capacity to start a physiological reaction inside the ECS, its frequently used to treat osteoporosis and joint pain; and may possibly expand the adequacy of some enemy of malignant growth drugs.

- **Clove oil:** A strong segment of clove oil is eugenol a ground-breaking cell reinforcement, mitigating, antimicrobial, and energizer. Beta-caryophyllene in cloves is a huge phytocannabinoid that can tie with CB2 receptors to diminish torment and irritation.

- **Echinacea:** You may be progressively familiar with echinacea as a virus cure, but this groundbreaking herb can also actuate CB1 receptors. It contains a compound called N-alkyl amides that are essentially the same as the effect of THC on torment, resistant framework, and irritation.

- **Peony:** This local bloom of China is an incredible wellspring of cannabinoids. Otherwise called peonia root, it is known for its capacity to decrease irritation in gout and other joint ailments, just as quieting muscle fits.

Appropriate Alternatives for Rick Simpson Hemp Oil

You may have known about Rick Simpson hemp oil. an oil that is fundamental from cannabis blossoms, it truly is high in the cannabinoid tetrahydrocannabinol (THC) and, as per Rick Simpson and others that are numerous has treated their malignant growth.

Does it truly work? Episodic proof clearly tips for the explanation that way. Unfortuitously, because of the shame cannabis that is encompassing cannabis, barely any medical research reports have endeavored. This is surely quickly changing, anyway for the present, there's definitely no unmistakable arrangement.

The Story of Rick Simpson Hemp Oil

Rick Simpson is extremely A canadian specialist who endured awful damage that offered him ringing that is consistent with the ears. The ailment genuinely influenced their disposition, their ability to center, alongside his life. None with respect to the medicines specialists recommended worked. an episode of *The Nature of Things* that talked concerning the potential that is medical of incited Rick Simpson to concentrate oil through the plant to use to manage their disease. In spite of the fact that the ringing was by and by here, the oil previously got it down intensely to a useful degree. He had been in a situation to rest by and by, his inconvenience wound up being under wraps, and along these lines had been their pulse levels. Rick Simpson recovered his life right.

A few years after the fact, Rick found three spots on their skin which were analyzed as epidermis malignant growth tumors. One spot had been precisely disposed of, together with the other two had been to be killed some time. As Rick Simpson recovered, he reviewed a 1974 news report that referenced the aftereffects of THC on malignant growth tumors cells in mice. He endeavored the oil on his two staying spots, and multiple times they surely were gone. When the malignant growth that was killed returned two or after three weeks, he oversaw it as a result of the oil, and again his skin had been recuperated.

Rick Simpson wanted the entire globe to get some answers concerning their finding and began offering his oil for nothing out of pocket to malignant growth tumors exploited people. Various were recuperated. Unfortuitously, numerous specialists when you take a gander at the medical field responded contrarily to Rick Simpson's story. at long last ready to give their story to a more extensive group of spectators at whatever point movie producer Christian Laurette made a narrative *Go Through the Cure* about Rick Simpson's life finding. The narrative incited research by Spanish researchers on people groups disease tumors patients that broke down the consequences of THC on malignancy tumors cells. found that THC had assaulted the malignant growth tumors cells while making the tissue that is healthy it unblemished. In any case, Rick Simpson hemp oil keeps on being perhaps not proper spots, not just since it contains THC since it is gotten from cannabis, at the same time, the psychoactive fixing in the plant. Another elective that is legal cannabidiol.

Cannabidiol and Cancer

Cannabidiol (CBD) could be the other cannabinoid that is major in cannabis blooms. In contrast to THC, CBD simply is not psychoactive and it is getting used to managing youthful ones with obstinate epilepsy. CBD additionally experiences lower levels of medical research, however basically like research encompassing THC, the measure of studies is expanding, and introductory discoveries are ensuring. We at present comprehend that CBD can slow the advancement of and limit its forcefulness, it might truly be more advantageous than THC. Like its psychoactive cousin, CBD had been found to keep healthy bosom tissue unblemished. Other research reports have found that CBD is successful against prostate disease tumors and lung malignancy.

Legal Sources of Cannabidiol

Not absolutely a wide range of cannabidiol fits in many states. CBD acquired from medical marijuana suitable in states where medical cannabis it self is legal. Regardless, it could be expelled from mechanical hemp, prompting oil that contains for all intents and purposes no THC. This oil is "hemp is approved to be utilized being a nourishment added substance by the FDA into the United states and can be gotten legally and used countrywide.

LAWS AND REGULATIONS ON MEDICINAL CANNABIS AROUND THE WORLD

As indicated by the INCB, the licit utilization of cannabis has expanded significantly since 2000. From that point forward, an ever increasing number of nations have begun to utilize cannabis and additionally cannabis extricates for medical purposes, notwithstanding logical research. In 2000, all out production was 1.3 tons; by 2015, it had expanded to 100.2 tons. Revealed necessities for 2017 demonstrate further development to almost 160 tons. The current encounters of setting up approaches empowering access to therapeutic cannabis are shifted and the various procedures that prompted these strategies can for the most part be arranged as pursues:

- Individual cases safeguarded in the courts which set points of reference, or sentences that are applied for the most part, similar to the case in Mexico and Canada

- Direct just procedures, for example, referenda and prominent discussions like in a few US states

- Legislative and open approach procedures drove by national or sub-national governments, as in Uruguay and different US states

- Companies were creating therapeutic cannabis and requesting that administration specialists encourage their licit use, for instance in the UK.

Logical Audit Of Cannabis By The United Nations

Aside from the basic leadership process, different elements can impact the sort and effect of the different administrative encounters. These incorporate the sort of society wherein the cannabis discussion happens, the level of improvement of its instructive and scholastic foundations, the quantity of experts devoted to considering the issue, the presence of a composed common society, the verifiable and social association with the plant, regardless of whether there are zones where cannabis is as of now being delivered in a nation, interest for cannabis and its subordinates for restorative or remedial purposes, and the open approach objectives sought after.

This can clarify the wide scope of reactions from nations to the interest for restorative cannabis use, which might be monetarily liberal like in the United States, or significantly statist on account of Uruguay (where open foundations handle all exercises identified with the production, preparing and closeout of cannabis). The encounters likewise vary with respect to characterizing restorative use, the sorts of products considered as medicines (for instance, a few nations just approve pharmaceuticals, for example, Sativex, while others permit home grew or non-pharmacological arrangements), regardless of whether development for individual use or the utilization of salves and oils is allowed, and so on. It is additionally important here that, even in instances of therapeutic guidelines, different types of cannabis use stay denied, with its hallowed utilize just permitted in Jamaica and recreational utilize just allowed in Uruguay and some US states. At last, different nations are at the underlying phase of the exchange, with proposed enactment viable in Costa Rica, Cyprus, Lithuania, Luxemburg, New Zealand, Saint Vincent and the Grenadines and South Africa.

Latin America And The Caribbean: New Pioneers In Therapeutic Cannabis Change

Latin America is at present the world chief in the advancement and appropriation of strategies enabling access to cannabis for helpful employments. Uruguay is the main nation on the planet to totally legalize the cannabis advertises for medical and logical purposes, just as for modern and recreational use. In this little nation, the state with help from the Institute for the Regulation and Control of Cannabis figures out who can create cannabis, just as how much and who can devour it, under which conditions. From one perspective, the administrative system for recreational use depends on giving licenses to people keen on planting, developing, collecting, delivering and commercializing cannabis, and incorporates a few types of access: self-development for individual use, cannabis clubs or buy in drug stores. These are totally unrelated, and the measure of cannabis that can be gained is constrained to 40g a month. On the other hand, the administrative framework for helpful cannabis sadly keeps on confronting different difficulties, including the way that the Ministry of Public Health does not approve the residential closeout of therapeutic cannabis.

Thus, patients wishing to get to restorative cannabis can just secure it inside the framework made for recreational purposes (that is, by delivering it themselves or getting to/buying a product that has not experienced all the logical testing vital for a medicine). An individual requiring treatment with Sativex or Marinol must demand an orange remedy (the most confined solution) and round out an application routed to the Ministry of Public Health to acquire the consent to import the product from abroad. In the event that the application is acknowledged, the expense of the product remains amazingly high. The Chilean case is unique, in spite of the fact that somehow or another like the Uruguayan experience. Despite the fact that there was no change of law twenty-thousand patients requiring restorative cannabis can get to it by means of medical solutions (Decree eight-four of the Institute for Public Health). In unique conditions, cannabis-based drugs can be approved for import, applications must be sent to the health authority taking care of enlistments.

The administrative organization is called ANAMED (Agencia Nacional del Medicamiento). As the drug stays difficult to reach in drug stores, the medical remedy can be utilized as a legal avocation of restorative use in court, which is permitted under article 4 of Law twenty-thousand. This empowers patients to develop plants at home (no predefined number) or to be an individual from an aggregate cannabis development club, inasmuch as the last is directed under law twenty-thousand and five-hundred on non-benefit resident cooperation. What is more, an undertaking drove by the Daya Foundation, related to the University of Valparaiso, Farmacopea Chilena and Knop Laboratories, expects to build up a phyto pharmaceutical that would be financially available.

Different nations, for example, Colombia, have likewise gained some ground. Law 1787, affirmed in 2015, made an administrative system for medical and logical access to cannabis, inside which the state holds command over the market and awards licenses to private elements for production, make, fare, change and research.66 When setting up the new administrative structure, the administration contemplated the way that cannabis was at that point being developed by subsistence ranchers in certain locales of Colombia and the law solicitations authorized makers to purchase their crude material legitimately from these little cultivators. This is a significant move to join the requirements of existing little scale cannabis ranchers in the new arrangement system. Be that as it may, specialized help is required for little cultivators to have the option to create crops that meet the necessary criteria for therapeutic cannabis.

Medicines created are phyto pharmaceuticals and can be gotten in approved drug stores, without a medical solution. The administration will expect to set a value that ensures access for all. Colombia is at present the nation that has enlisted the most elevated restorative cannabis yield with the INCB for 2018. In Jamaica, cannabis for therapeutic or remedial purposes must be suggested or endorsed by an enrolled doctor or a health expert guaranteed by the Ministry of Health. The import of cannabis products by patients is permitted as long as the doctor guarantees that the patient is experiencing a disease. In any case, not many experts endorse cannabis as a medicine. Visitors or individuals who don't dwell in

Jamaica can apply for a license that enables them to buy and have up to two ounces (56g) of ganja. To do as such, they should display a specialist's solution or sign a willful announcement expressing their medical condition. With the primary approvals dating from 2014, Brazil has since permitted the importation of prescriptions dependent on CBD oil, including THC and marijuana blossoms in 2016, for medical and restorative use.

In any case, the Brazilian Federal Medical Board disallows the medicine by specialists of marijuana in its vegetal structure, under extraordinary conditions. Import requires consistence with a progression of necessities set up by the National Health Surveillance Agency (Agencia Nacional de Vigilancia Sanitaria, ANVISA). These incorporate patients' enrollment, taking care of managerial systems for import face to face, and applying for a license from the office. The probability of self-development of cannabis for such purposes stays under exchange. Argentina, Peru and Mexico have additionally embraced other, less aspiring, administrative procedures. In those nations, changes came about because of dynamic weight from common society and patients' gatherings, prompting the endorsement of approaches considering the deal and utilization of therapeutic cannabis. In October 2017, Peru endorsed its *Law directing the restorative and remedial utilization of cannabis and its subsidiaries* which was marked by President Pablo Kuczynski on sixteenth November.

The law presents the utilization of libraries for the different gatherings who wish to get to cannabis (for example patients, shippers, research elements and open substances), and an arrangement of government licenses for research, importation, commercialization and production. It is significant that the nation has perceived the advantages of cannabis for the treatment of indications brought about by infections, for example, disease or numerous cases of sclerosis. In any case, the administrative system that will guarantee legal access to the substance stays to be explained. In Argentina, then, a standard was given that enables patients to import their prescription while the state starts the nearby production of pharmaceuticals for the domestic market.

In Mexico, the changes to the General Health Law and the Criminal Code in 2017 presently permit the utilization of cannabis for medical and logical purposes. The Ministry of Health was requested to give an open arrangement on the issue to guarantee that patients approach pharmacological products with and without THC. At long last, Bolivia is the most recent Latin American nation to date to have revised its medication enactment to permit therapeutic cannabis. Concurred inside the casing work of a more extensive medication enactment embraced on sixteenth March20 17, people and organizations must enlist and demand an earlier approval to the Ministry of Health for the import, fare, exchange or production of therapeutic cannabis. Extraordinary and restricted approvals may likewise be allowed by the Ministry of Health for research on restorative cannabis.

North America: Pioneer In The Medicinal Cannabis Industry

The United States and Canada might be the most exceptional nations in the advancement of a therapeutic cannabis industry. In the United States, twenty-nine states directly have an authorization allowing remedial cannabis use, similarly as the advancement, production, getting ready, arrangement and assessment gathering of cannabis and its subordinates. The United States is in this way a genuine case of blended procedures in with blended outcomes where the two choices and administrative procedures reacted to various needs and interests, mirroring an intriguing mixture of administrative systems that sway between those organizing general health and those seeking after real business finishes and income producing objectives:

- 14 states have legalized restorative cannabis by choice: California in 1996; Washington, Oregon and Alaska in 1998; Maine in 1999; Nevada, Hawaii and Colorado in 2000; Montana in 2004;

Michigan in 2008; Arizona in 2010; and North Dakota, Florida and Arkansas in 2016

- 15 states have taken the administrative course: Vermont in 2004; Rhode Island in 2006; New Mexico in 2007; New Jersey in 2010; Delaware in 2011; Massachusetts and Connecticut in 2012; New Hampshire and Illinois in 2013; Nueva York, Minnesota and Maryland in 2014; Pennsylvania and Ohio in 2016; and West Virginia in 2017.In Canada, there are around 44 authorized makers approved by the Ministry of Health, just as a large number of Canadians authorized to have and expend therapeutic cannabis. In the two cases, self-development is permitted insofar as it does not surpass six plants and use can be defended.

Europe: Positive However Constrained Advances

In Europe, close by entrenched models of therapeutic cannabis as in the Netherlands, the previous year has seen the appropriation of different restorative cannabis plans, specifically in Greece, Poland and Slovenia.

Different nations have been increasingly mindful, concentrating solely on pilot ventures. The Netherlands, in the mean time, legalized the restorative utilization of cannabis in 2000, and made the Bureau for Medicinal Cannabis (BMC) making a solid pharmacological industry, driven by Bedrocan Medical Cannabis which has the imposing business model of all therapeutic cannabis production and conveyance. All cannabis going through the BMC is created by Bedrocan which created and institutionalized residential interest and fare a portion of the five sorts of pharmaceutical cannabis flos (blossom) prescriptions arranged with various rates of THC and CBD. Therapeutic cannabis is delivered across the nation and constrained by the Medicinal Cannabis Agency. It tends to be acquired in drug stores for various pathologies, just when the patient is in control of a medical remedy.

Restorative use has expanded significantly over the previous decade, with more than 50,000 patients presently being recommended cannabis in the Netherlands. Germany has quite recently finished the authoritative changes important to grow the medical utilization of cannabis. Under the watchful eye of the new law that went in January 2017, patients could just access medical cannabis through a unique singular approval. Germany is currently one of the main nations on the planet to incorporate medical cannabis in the fundamental scope of meds that must be secured by both private safety net providers and open health services. A national Cannabis Agency was set up under the Federal Institute for Drugs and Medical Devices (BfArM) to supervise the new procedure, as recommended by the global medication settlements. The 2017 law likewise permits the improvement of residential production of cannabis, despite the fact that until further notice all cannabis meds proceed with imported, basically from the Netherlands.

Somewhere else in Europe, an absence of essential guidelines of therapeutic cannabis in nations like the United Kingdom and the Czech Republic has hampered access to these prescriptions for a huge number of patients. In the previous, the administration just allows the utilization of Sativex for patients with various cases of sclerosis, under medical remedy. The general health administration in the United Kingdom has additionally settled that each patient must compensation for their prescription, at the expense of about 500 Euros a month. In the Czech Republic, despite the fact that the nation legalized medical cannabis in 2013, there is an atomic procedure for obtaining licenses to create, sell or buy products got from cannabis. There keeps on being vulnerability about the extension and capability of this change, both for the welfare of the patients and for the advancement of an industry that can add to the development in the accessible stockpile, which stays insufficient all through the mainland. As in the United Kingdom, the cost of the drug is additionally a significant test; since therapeutic cannabis isn't secured by the health protection framework. As expressed over, a few nations have as of late pushed forward with a change in the zone of therapeutic cannabis. In Poland, for instance, first November 2017 denoted the main day on which therapeutic cannabis could be sold in enrolled drug stores.

Patients need extraordinary consent from a local pharmaceutical investigator and a doctor certify by the

Ministry of Health. The law just permits the importation of cannabis (essentially from the Netherlands), as opposed to household production or self-development. Likewise, in Slovenia, as of February 2018, the Decree on the order of unlawful drugs (Official Gazette of the Republic of Slovenia, no. 45/14, 22/16 and 14/17) enables medical specialists to recommend cannabinoid-based drugs (manufactured, characteristic and the alleged therapeutic cannabis), just as institutionalized buds and blossoming highest points of cannabis (despite the fact that the last stays to be completely executed by and by). This arrangement change required moving cannabis from Group I to Group II in the rundown of illegal substances of Slovenia. The Ministry of Health is responsible for actualizing the therapeutic cannabis plot. On first March 2018 Greece received the bill 'Arrangements for the Production of final results of therapeutic cannabis'. It is vital that most of the parliamentary ideological groups bolstered the bill; in spite of the fact that resistance groups casted a ballot against the bill in the last vote.

The bill recommends that Greece's medical patients can get to therapeutic cannabis products, in acknowledgment of their advantages for explicit ailments. It additionally recommends that people can develop cannabis for the sole reason for delivering therapeutic cannabis products in the nation. At long last, the bill perceives the financial capability of therapeutic cannabis; with the making of new openings and the capability of sending out products to the universal market. At long last, in different nations, restorative cannabis is restricted to pilot ventures. In Denmark, for instance, cannabis for helpful designs is as yet illegal, however an experimental run program will start on first January 2018 for a predetermined number of patients with explicit health issues (for example various sclerosis, constant torment and sickness). Therapeutic cannabis additionally stays illegal in Ireland, however some pilot tasks are in progress, and a bill was passed by the Dail (Irish parliament) in December 2016, despite the fact that the law has not yet come into force.84Israel:

The Middle Eastern: Special Case

Today, there are more than fifty labs directing research on restorative cannabis in the different colleges and scholastic establishments of Israel. The thorough logical learning and investigation of chances for logical and modern advancement have driven Israel to attempt changes on cannabis that don't really coordinate with its methodology towards different drugs. The nation endorsed the therapeutic utilization of cannabis in 1992 and before long turned into an inside for logical research and improvement of cannabis assortments and mechanical products. The enactment is executed by an uncommonly settled unit in the Ministry of Health, the Israeli Agency on Medical Cannabis (IMCA), which set up a controlling advisory group in a joint effort with the Israeli police, the Ministry of Agriculture and the Ministry of Economy, headed by one of the logical pioneers of the field: Prof Meshulam.

The IMCA issues a few sorts of licenses for development, extraction and bundling plants, and dispersion. The IMCA is additionally answerable for the approval of uncommon clinicians who are permitted to recommend cannabis to patients experiencing extreme torment and various different side effects. Extra diseases can be treated in emergency clinics as a major aspect of clinical preliminaries. By 2017, somewhere in the range of 40,000 patients were getting therapeutic cannabis.

Asia:

Despite the fact that Asia keeps on being at the front line of severe medication strategies, and restorative cannabis stays disallowed in Japan, Vietnam, Pakistan, Cambodia and Nepal. Be that as it may, there have been certain advancements in a few nations of the area. In India, the law recognizes two sorts of cannabis products: ganja (the blooming or fruiting highest points of the cannabis plant) and charash or hashish (cannabisresin), with regulations being increasingly loose for the previous. The nation as of now has some legal arrangements for the restorative and logical utilization of the plant, however these arrangements presently can not seem to be actualized. Since 2017, different political figures, including Maneka Ghandi and MP Dr. Dharamvir Ghandi, demonstrated their help to cannabis strategy change. In the region of research on therapeutic cannabis, the 2015 Phyto pharmaceutical Act was passed to quicken examinations on plant-based medicines, a move that has the capability of pulling in speculations into cannabis research from huge organizations.

In the Philippines, while President Duterte kept on pursuing his war on drugs the nation over, the House Committee on Health endorsed the Medical Compassionate Medical Cannabis Act in September 2016. The law forbids the utilization of cannabis in its crude structure, and stipulates that patients need earlier approval from a specialist, and the treatment will be conveyed in committed focuses with a unique permit from the Department of Health, in clinics. The Philippine Drug Enforcement Agency is answerable for the guideline and regulation of restorative cannabis, which can be utilized to treat different diseases, including joint inflammation, epilepsy and numerous sclerosis, among others. The bill additionally plans to make a research office on therapeutic cannabis. In the interim, in Thailand an open discussion was held in August 2016 to expel cannabis from Category 5 of the nation's medication enactment, and the Agricultural Council was entrusted with building up a proposition for the decriminalization of the substance for thought by the legislature. From first January 2017, hemp was decriminalized in 15 areas and six territories of the northern district.

Oceania:

Australia gaining ground: There have been huge advancements in Australia on the therapeutic cannabis front as of late. Since 2016 the nation has another national body that can issue licenses to cultivators and direct restorative cannabis crops with the goal that therapeutic marijuana can be developed in Australia. Medical specialists may supply a restorative cannabis product to a patient in the wake of advising the pertinent administrative power and acquiring earlier authorization from the state or domain government division. This is done on a patient-by-tolerant premise and therapeutic cannabis can likewise be utilized for clinical preliminaries. Probably the most significant changes have happened at the state and region level. The territory of New South Wales originally induced wide-running therapeutic cannabis preliminaries and furnished the police with the power not to arraign critically ill patients utilizing cannabis for medical purposes.

Few kids with the most pessimistic scenario of medication inhabitant epilepsy can likewise be recommended restorative marijuana under a merciful access plot. Victoria was the principal state to set up a state-based therapeutic cannabis plan enabling youngsters with serious epilepsy to be given the medication. The entirety of different states and domains have plans to empower access to therapeutic cannabis through remedy for organizing of conditions. Queensland built up the primary direction reports for health professionals in March 2017. In December 2017, the Commonwealth delivered the national rules for five conditions and distributed these on the Therapeutic Goods Administration site. New Zealand likewise presented the Misuse of Drugs Amendment Bill in December 2017 with the objective of making restorative cannabis accessible without criminal obligation.

Contemplations For Legislative Reform

Among the nation models introduced above, there is a wide scope of instruments accessible to guarantee access to therapeutic cannabis:

- Unique individual licenses to import and utilize restorative cannabis, while keeping up generally denials over the plant, however setting up special cases to the law to guarantee patients' entrance to cannabis (for example in Poland).

- Guideline of supply through the formation of a permitting framework conceded to people or private substances as indicated by the kind of movement they participate in (production, fabricate, send out, handling, research, transport or deal), inside which the state can assume different jobs – from focal control to negligible assertion through administrative bodies (for example in Colombia or Peru).

- Guideline of interest with systems enabling legal access to prescriptions or natural cannabis arrangements through: self-development, cannabis clubs, postal requests, deal in facilities or deal in drug stores (for example in Uruguay for recreational, and as a matter of course, therapeutic use).

- The plan and usage of open approaches that manage access to specific products, in consistence with the administrative framework set up for medicines (for example in Germany). Contingent upon the kind of administrative system and to what extent it has been set up, different effects have been recognized on the ground notwithstanding the proof previously referenced above with respect to the health advantages of therapeutic cannabis:

- The fantasy around increments in illegal cannabis use as an immediate consequence of the usage of restorative cannabis administrative systems doesn't remain constant, particularly among youths for whom cannabis use commonness has stayed stable, in nations like the United States.

- Similarly, the quantity of auto collisions brought about by intense cannabis inebriation has not expanded perceptibly in purviews where the utilization of arrangements with THC or home grown types of cannabis is allowed.

- There have been no recorded passing's brought about by cannabis; despite what might be expected, the endurance rate and personal satisfaction of patients have improved.

There has been no sharp ascent in wrongdoing, maybe there is even proof in some US states executing a therapeutic cannabis plot that the wrongdoing rates have dropped by as much as 13%.

RECOMMENDATIONS

The data accessible so far makes it conceivable to plot the accompanying arrangement recommendations:

- Legalize cannabis for restorative use, just as meds and helpful substances got from cannabis, for all afflictions distinguished by logical research, and not exclusively constraining access for a couple of self-assertively decided diseases.

- Immediately incorporate drugs got from cannabis in the essential scope of medicines, that is, without the requirement for legal activities requiring the state to do as such, and keeping away from additionally the significant expenses that individual importation of such prescription would include for every particular case.

- Reform the essential laws to make and distribute a spending plan to guarantee the steady age of logical research.

- Coordinate every single pertinent organization to streamline the different specialized and clean procedures that enable new drugs to arrive at the market rapidly, while continually guaranteeing the most noteworthy potential models for purchaser health security.

- Establish the components important to keep away from the making of imposing business models or a limitation of the market to a couple of explicit gatherings who might hold all licenses and deal licenses to the inconvenience of the health and financial welfare of the overall public.

- Include the patients in basic leadership procedures identified with the improvement of general enactment and regulations, in order to set up standards that react to their needs with regards to every particular state.

- Avoid building up self-assertive ideas (for instance, the centralization of a specific psychoactive substance) that would influence access or result in the denial of a medicine that contains those substances.

- Offer specialized help to doctors, giving them the instruments they have to comprehend both the advantages and the health dangers of therapeutic cannabis.

- Implement government funded training and mindfulness raising efforts for the overall population and patients on restorative cannabis.

- Every authoritative measure ought to incorporate residential regulations for production, instead of being restricted to the importation of products. The subsequent administrative systems ought to likewise consider all estimates important to advance the incorporation of existing little scale producers and, to the extent that conceivable, do as such under conditions equivalent or progressively ideal to those conceded to new allow holders and additionally capital-serious remote industry.

- Small-scale ranchers associated with cannabis development for subsistence purposes ought to be engaged with the basic leadership procedures to empower the joining of their needs, and ought to get specialized help so they can take an interest in the 'matter' of therapeutic cannabis.

CONCLUSION

The way that Cannabis Pharmacy oil is free from the psychoactive THC compound, is the thing that, makes the products so engaging. For quite a long time, marijuana has been thought to give individuals health benefits. Be that as it may, the issue was that it was incomprehensible or testing to confine the psychoactive THC fixing from the health-giving cannabinoids. Cannabis Pharmacy oil is a superb, ease, low-reaction path for individuals to discover alleviation from certain health conditions without the mind-changing impacts of THC, or standard pharmaceutical drugs, which can accompany a large group of unfavorable, troubling symptoms. It is an all-common product, where the cannabinoids are separated from the hemp plant. The cannabinoids are then weakened with transporter oil, the most well-known being coconut oil or hemp seed oil. CBD oil represents cannabidiol, and it is a characteristic, expanding prevalent product utilized for treating a large group of illnesses, throbs, and agonies Cannabis Pharmacy oil comes in two primary sorts.

The principal type is made out of confined cannabinoids, while the subsequent kind is "wide range" CBD oil that envelops different parts present in the marijuana plant. The marijuana plant Cannabis Sativa has in excess of 100 substance mixes known as cannabinoids. These cannabinoids are what give CBD oil its capacity to mend and ease torment and other basic health issues. It's imperative to comprehend that the dynamic cannabinoids in CBD oil are not equivalent to THC or tetrahydrocannabinol. THC is the compound in the marijuana plant that makes an individual vibe "high." CBD, nonetheless, isn't psychoactive and can't make somebody high and is gotten from the governmentally authorized modern hemp plant. All in all, the advantages of CBD oil are utilized to treat a scope of constant illnesses, most quite ceaseless agony, joint pain, and nervousness. The advantages of CBD oil are not successful in treating intense diseases, or extreme health issues.

CANNABIS
COOKBOOK

By

DOREEN WEED

© Copyright 2020 Doreen Weed

All rights reserved.

Table of Contents

INTRODUCTION TO CANNABIS 13

MODERN HERBAL MEDICINE 17

CANNABIS HISTORY, PROPERTIES AND PRODUCTS 34

MEDICAL CANNABIS: 55

HOW TO CHOOSE AND USE 55

CANNABIS PHENOTYPE AND GENOTYPE 68

CANNABIS STRAINS 77

DIFFERENCE BETWEEN THC AND CBD STRAINS 82

PRODUCTION OF CANNABIS PHARMACY OIL 109

CANNABIS PHARMACY OILS AND ITS USAGE 123

USEFULNESS OF CANNABIS OIL FOR THE AGED 142

CANNABIS PHARMACY OIL ON PETS 148

NEGATIVE IMPLICATIONS OF CANNABIS ABUSE ON GENERAL AND ORAL HEALTH 156

RELATED EFFECTS ON USAGE OF CANNABIS PHARMACY OIL 161

IS ALL CANNABIS OIL THE SAME? 180

ALTERNATIVES TO CANNABIS PHARMACY OIL 192

LAWS AND REGULATIONS ON MEDICINAL CANNABIS AROUND THE WORLD 200

RECOMMENDATIONS 225

CONCLUSION 229

WHAT IS CANNABIS..242

How to recognize marijuana CBD and THC 244

HISTORY OF CANNABIS 246

Hemp for food...259

Hemp for health & body 259

Hemp for Fuel 260

The controversy of classifying: hemp vs cannabis...260

Hemp seed oil and hemp extract vs cannabis oil 261

HOW CANNABIS BENEFITS WOMEN'S GYNECOLOGICAL HEALTH 262

WHAT IS CANNABIS STRESS?............................266

Different kinds of strains..................................268

THE STEP–UP TECHNIQUE 274

Palm Mincer 275

So, How Much CBD Should You Take? 276

TCheck Dosage Checker 276

What's the Right Dose of CBD?.....................276

EXPANDING LAWS 277

Volcano Vaporizer.......................................277

Fruity Pebbly...277

CANNABIS DOSING GUIDE 278

Macro (Or Therapeutic) Dose........................278

Standard Dose...279

HOW TO CALCULATE EDIBLE POTENCY.................. 280

General Dosage Guidelines........................... 281

Regularly talk to a medical care expert 281

HEMP SEEDS FOR WEIGHT LOSS........................... 283

HEMP HEARTS VS HEMP SEEDS 284

Understand CBD as well as THC Contents ... 286

Just how exactly hemp seeds support weight loss? 288

Best ways to lose weight with cannabis seeds........ 293

SOME BENEFITS OF HEMP SEEDS 295

HOW TO MAKE CSB BROWNIES.............................. 299

Non-Vegan CBD brownie..................................... 299

Vegan CBD Brownies.. 301

CBD brownies with vaped buds 302

CBD brownies with Cannabis butter 302

CANNABIS COCKTAIL SYRUPS 303

Thai High 303

SIP IT UP 304

Smoke with Spices. 304

Lime wedge to prepare 304

WANDERER.. 305

Marijuana Milk (sugar-free). 305

Vanilla Cannabis Milkshake. 306

STRAWBERRY CANNA-BASIL LEMONADE...............307

Marijuana Thai Iced Tea...............308

Cup Of Unsweetened Cocoa Powder....................308

Hot Canna-Buttered Apple Cider.......................309

Sparkling Pear Prosecco Canna Punch..................310

Cannabis Olive Oil....................................311

HOW TO MAKE STONER SWEETS 313

POT CHEF...314

VINAIGRETTE.......................................314

STUFFED STONED JALAPEÑO POPPERS 315

SATIVA SHRIMP SPRING ROLLS WITH MANGO SAUCE.
....317

MARIJUANA GUACAMOLE 319

MINI KIND VEGGIE BURRITOS 320

PICO DE GANJA AND NACHOS.............................322

BRUSCHETTA..323

KIND BUD BRUSCHETTA WITH POT PESTO 324

Marijuana Pancakes..324

MEAT LOAF 325

Cannabis Spinach 326

Marijuana Baked Salmon.................................. 327

Marijuana Joe Sandwiches 327

Cannabis Balsamic Vinaigrette........................ 328

Sautéed squash.. 329

Marijuana Spaghetti...................................... 329

Marijuana Pepper and Artichoke Dip 330

CANNABIS POTATO AND OLIVE OIL SOUP 331

Cannabis Alfredo Pasta Sauce.......................... 331

Marijuana Chili.. 332

Cannabis Turkey Stuffing................................ 333

Cannabis Caesar Salad................................... 334

Marijuana Crab Stuffed Mushrooms...................... 335

Marijuana Flour. 336

Cannabis Olivia 336

Cannabis Fried Butter Ball 337

Marijuana pie N Chicken 338

Potatoe Mash. 339

CANNABIS PIZZA 340

Cannabis Salsa N Papaya 341

Cannabis Salmon.. 342

Marijuana Salmon Mapple 343

Marijuana Tilapia Tacos.................................. 344

Baked Cannabis Tilapia 345

Cannabis Hash Brown Casserole 345

Marijuana Baked Pizza Sandwich 346

Marijuana BBQ Beef Sandwiches 347

Marijuana Basil Chicken Pasta............................348

Cannabis Basil Shrimp Pasta..............................349

Cannabis Tea...350

CANNABIS SHOTS-JELLO. 352

Marijuana Cupcakes 353

Cannabis Brownies 354

BUTTER 356

Cannabis Apple Pecan Galaxy Cake 357

Cannabis Chocolate Pudding...............................357

Cannabis Cashew Cookies..................................358

Cannabis Sugar Cookie....................................359

Velvet Cupcakes 360

Marijuana Oatmeal Cookies. 361

Canna Lemon Bread 361

Orange Cake..362

Chocolate Milkshake......................................363

Banana Blueberry Healthy Smoothie.......................363

Cinnamon Coffee Cake 364

Canna Flat Bread.. 365

Tiramisu Milk Shake 366

Cannabis Bread.. 367

Canna Extra Pound Cake 367

Marijuana scones.. 368

Sugar Squares 369

Delicious Chocolate Space Cake 370

Marijuana Cheesecake 371

Marijuana Truffles... 372

Chocolate Chip Cookies.. 373

Cannabis Pumpkin Muffins..................................... 374

Marijuana Orange Dark Chocolate Chip Cookies 375

Marijuana Cranberry and also Macadamia Nut Cookies
.... 376

Health Bars 377

Marijuana Caramel Walnut Dream Bars................. 378

Iced Marshmallow Cookies..................................... 378

Marijuana Brown-eyes 379

Marijuana Peanut Butter Cup Cookies 380

Marijuana Butterscotch Space Pops 381

CONCLUSION.. 383

What's the meaning of cannabis?

Cannabis describes a group of three plants with psychoactive skills: *Cannabis sativa, Cannabis indica* and *Cannabis ruderalis*.

When the blossoms of these plants are harvested and dried out, you are entrusted to among the most usual medications in the world. Some call it to weed, and some call it *pot*, and also others call it cannabis.

Toda more and more people are making use of the term marijuana to refer to weed. Others feel it is more neutral contrasted to terms like weed or pot, which some people still connect with its unlawful use.

Cannabis is typically consumed for its relaxing as well as soothing results. Clinical marijuana is utilised to treat the signs and symptoms of problems instead than as a treatment for the condition itself.

A few of the problems that clinical marijuana has been approved to deal with in lots of states consist of:

- AIDS
- Alzheimer's illness
- Cancer
- Crohn's condition
- Eating disorders
- Glaucoma
- Cachexia
- Migraine headaches
- Seizures

- Extreme discomfort
- Severe nausea
- Consistent muscle spasms
- Losing disease

Additional research study on the prospective advantages of medical marijuana is recurring. Recognised, as well as legitimately sanctioned use cannabis for the therapy or relief of signs, will undoubtedly continue to evolve as scientists check out these uses.

Since 2019, medical marijuana is legal in thirty-three states in addition to Washington, D.C

What to know about marijuana use

Pot describes the dried out fallen leaves, stems, flowers, as well as seeds from the hemp plant Cannabis. The main active component in cannabis is the mind-altering chemical delta-9-tetrahydrocannabinol (THC).

Marijuana is one of the most common illegal drug used in the United States. According to a national study on substance abuse and wellness from 2017, concerning 45% of Americans over the age of twelve have used cannabis.

As of the 2018 midterm elections, ten states as well as Washington DC had legislated cannabis for entertainment usage for adults over twenty-one years-old. Over thirty countries have regulations on guides legislating marijuana for medical use only, while numerous others have only legalised oils with low-THC content. Cannabis is still unlawful under federal law.

It is additionally known As There are over 200-slang-terms for cannabis, including pot, natural herb, weed, yard, widow, boom, marijuana, hash, Mary Jane, marijuana, bubble periodontal, northern lights, fruity juice, gangster, Afghani, skunk, and persistent.

Drug Class: Marijuana is usually classified as a depressant, although it additionally has stimulant as well as hallucinogenic residential properties.

Common Side Effects: Side impacts of cannabis usage consist of modified senses, state of mind changes, difficulty assuming, as well as impaired memory. In high dosages, it can prompt hallucinations, psychosis, and deceptions.

How to recognize marijuana CBD and THC

Cannabis resembles a shredded, green-brown mix of plant products. However, it can look varies depending on exactly how it is ready or packaged.

Each has its results and also utilises: Each has its results and also utilises:

CBD. It is a non-psychoactive cannabinoid, suggesting it will not obtain you *high*. It is typically used to help reduce inflammation as well as convenience pain. It likewise assists with nausea, migraine headaches, seizures, and also anxiety. Scientists are still attempting to recognise the effectiveness of their clinical usage ultimately.

THC. It is the primary psychedelic substance in marijuana. THC is in charge of the *high* that the majority of people connect with pot.

Uncover out more about the differences between THC and CBD.

In the Ancient World, hemp was a usual farming crop collected for its high-protein seeds, oil, as well as fibre-uses for rope and garments. Hemp is one selection of the Cannabis plant, but it does not have the same mind-altering impacts as marijuana.

In Ancient China and somewhere else in the globe, nevertheless, hemp was grown for food and also had hundreds of various other usages so it was only all-natural for people to discover that different types of the Cannabis plant can be made use of medicinally. In ancient times, marijuana was used to reduce discomfort and deal with various conditions.

The short-term results of cannabis can also differ based on your method of consumption. If you smoke marijuana, you will feel the effects win some minutes. Yet if you by mouth consume something, such as a tincture, food, or pill product, it might be several hours before you feel anything.

Marijuana usually comes in various pressures. These hang classifications used to show the effects of different marijuana products.

Below you can find a primer on some common strains and also their possible impacts.

- Relaxation
- Giddiness

- Experiencing points around you, such as views and audios, more intensely
- enhanced appetite

Transformed assumption of time and events, these effects are frequently minimal in items consisting of really high levels of CBD compared to THC.

These impacts are much less usual in items containing more CBD than THC.

Medieval doctors mixed the plant right into teas or medicines to treat discomfort and even other disorders; at that time, it had not been a very controlled compound the way it is today, where in the U.S. it's listed as a Schedule I drug along with LSD and also heroin. Here is a brief history of clinical marijuana to much better understand the level of its efficiency in treatments as well as therapies.

A brief history of medical marijuana: from Ancient anesthesia to the modern dispensary

For years in U.S.A. marijuana has been painted as the hallucinogen of hippies and also stoners who lay around smoking cigarettes dope to the detriment of their cognitive function.

In 2737 B.C. According to Chinese tale, Emperor Shen Neng was among the first significant leaders in the old globe to officially prescribe marijuana tea to treat numerous health problems including gout pain, rheumatism, jungle fever, as well as poor memory, according to Understanding Cannabis: A Makeover at the Scientific Proof.

In states where clinical marijuana got legalised, there seems to be basic agreement that it's reasonably practical in treating a selection of ailments. One 2014 research study discovered that over 90% of individuals in California that were recommended marijuana reported that it helped them deal with a severe clinical problem.

Compared to the Western world and also other parts of Asia like China and even Japan, India had always continued to be very closely tied to marijuana use medicinally, religiously, recreationally, and mentally. Marijuana was as well as continues to be mixed into unique beverages that are made use of for essential satisfaction yet likewise for medical factors. Among the most preferred of these beverages is bhang-- a mix of marijuana paste (made from the buds as well as leaves), milk, ghee, as well as flavours.

Later, the Indian Hemp Drugs Commission defined the history as well as the culture of marijuana in India: *"To the Hindu the hemp plant is divine. A guardian stays in the bhang fallen leave. To see in a desire the fallen leaves, plant, or water of bhang is fortunate. No excellent thing can involve the man who steps underfoot the holy bhang fallen leave. A longing for bhang foretells joy. Besides as a treatment for fever, bhang has numerous medical virtues. It remedies dysentery and sunstroke, removes phlegm, accelerates digestion, sharpens hunger, makes the tongue of the lisper plain, freshens the intellect, and provides performance to the body and also gaiety to the mind."* While at the time there was most likely little clinical evidence behind the medical usefulness of weed, it shows that the drug had been mostly 1550 B.C. Ancient Egypt's Ebers Papyrus makes a note of clinical cannabis as a means to treat inflammation.

In the fourth book of the Vedas, called the Atharvaveda which implies *Science of Charms*, ancient Indian writers refer to bhang as one of the *"Five kingdoms of natural herbs which release us from anxiety."* Later, as the beverage ended up being a lot more prominent, it was defined as having the ability to make individuals satisfied, warm, and enhance *mental powers* along with *remove wind as well as phlegm.*

In 100 A.D, in China, the Shennong Bencaojing, a clinical publication, describes marijuana as dama (da meaning great and ma meaning marijuana) as well as notes that the blossoms, the seeds, and the leaves of the plant can be beneficial in medicine.

In 200 A.D, Hua Tuo, a Chinese doctor, is the first tape-recorded physician to use cannabis as an anesthetic throughout the surgical treatment. Throughout this time, Chinese physicians likewise utilized the origin, leaves, and also oil of marijuana to deal with blood clots, tapeworms, irregularity, and even hair loss.

CONTEMPORARY

During 1500s the Spanish brought marijuana to South America, but throughout the North American colonization, there was just hemp made use of for functional objectives like clothing, bagging, paper, and also ropes for the maritime industry. The hemp market largely relied upon slave labor, as well as cannabis had not been introduced to America as a medical or psychoactive medicine up until years later.

In the late 1700s some American clinical journals were suggesting using hemp seeds as well as origins to treat numerous health problems, including skin inflammation and also urinary incontinence. William O'Shaughnessy was an Irish medical professional in the British East India Company who promoted medical cannabis's advantages for rheumatism and queasiness in England and also America.

MEDIEVAL

Throughout the Middle Ages, cannabis was a commonly preferred drug between the East. Due to the fact that red wine was forbidden in Islam, numerous Muslims looked to smoke hashish the Arab word for marijuana likewise called "turf. It was likewise used in traditional Arabic medicine. incorporated in clinical life in India for countless years.

Around 100-1000s A.D, all through the Middle Ages in Europe, marijuana may not have been a spiritual or religious hallucinogen like it remained in India, but it was still integrated into herbal remedies. Hemp is used to treating tumors, cough, as well as jaundice. Surprisingly enough, middle ages medical professionals as well as herbalists still warned of utilizing cannabis exceedingly-- believing that excessive could trigger sterility as well as other harmful problems.

In 1906 the U.S. Food and also Drug Administration (FDA) is developed to avoid another morphine addiction situation as many individuals were becoming addicted to opium, morphine, and heroin, which weren't correctly regulated. The FDA generally managed opium and morphine throughout this time, and not a lot of cannabis, however its production indicated a huge shift in drug policy in America.

During this time around, Mexican immigrants going into the U.S. introduced marijuana to the nation (as well as words cannabis itself likely come from Mexico), popularizing the recreational use of the medication more. However, several Americans saw those who smoked weed as problematic and also debaucherous, linking marijuana with lower class criminality.

In 1914 the substance abuse, under the Harrison Act, is officially proclaimed a criminal activity.

The government likewise passes the Marihuana Tax Act, making the usage of non-medical weed illegal. Marijuana was still utilized in numerous medical treatments, albeit in controlled types.

In 1970 marijuana was classified as a Schedule of drug together with even more hazardous ones, and also was provided as having no approved medical use. Despite the fact that some early American clinical journals had actually started listing the clinical uses of marijuana, the government limited any kind of additional research right into it until much more recently.

this time, Chinese physicians likewise utilized the origin, leaves, and also oil of marijuana to deal with blood clots, tapeworms, irregularity, and even hair loss.

DIFFERENCE BETWEEN MEDICAL MARIJUANA AND RECRETIONAL MARIJUANA STOCK

Medical marijuana is a type of therapy prescribed by medical professionals for a wide variety of health and wellness problems and also signs. Because of this, a client needs to receive a prescription before he or she can obtain accessibility to cannabis therapy. Today, the medication has been made use of to treat Alzheimer's, different kinds of cancer cells, numerous mental wellness conditions, multiple sclerosis, queasiness, and pain.

Medicines that integrate cannabis might find significant applications in government health care. A 2016 term paper by Ashley Bradford as well as W. David Bradford from the University of Georgia located that prescription drug sales for painkillers dropped considerably in states which legislated clinical cannabis. *"National total reductions in Medicare program and enrollee investing when states implemented clinical cannabis legislation were approximated to be $165.2 million each year in 2013"* wrote the authors.

Clinical marijuana has been legislated by more than thirty states in some style (as of May 2019). The Food, as well as Drug Administration (FDA), has accepted four medicines with chemicals from or similar to the ones found in the cannabis plant, consisting of Epidiolex, a medication utilised to deal with an extreme as well as rare kind of epilepsy in youngsters.

While research study right into medical cannabis is still restricted due to restrictions avoiding researchers from acquiring the drug, recent studies have discovered some restorative elements of medical cannabis. As an example, a 2015 study located that marijuana could be reliable in dealing with schizophrenia. Research study has additionally shown that it can help recover busted bones, quit extreme seizures, and also cure migraines. And also one 2014 research recommended that marijuana might be reliable in targeting mind tumours, though much more research is needed to reproduce those outcomes.

Since April 2015, twenty-three states in the U.S. have legislated medical cannabis, yet just people with particular certifications can acquire it. That will normally require kids with epileptic problems, or often cancer cells patients that use cannabis to relieve the side effects of chemotherapy or radiation. Some states allow people with HIV/AIDs, Parkinson's disease, numerous sclerosis, or perhaps Crohn's condition to get medical marijuana.

Which has been circulating as some type of therapy for thousands of years around the globe, they're possibly right.

In spite of this, the market has been moving forward. A research study carried out in 2018 stated that Sanofis Aventis (SNA) and also Merck (MRK) are amongst the leading cannabis-related patent owners. As well as companies presently involved in using cannabis for clinical usages are GW Pharmaceuticals (GWPH), Tilray (TLRY), Corbus Pharmaceuticals (CRBP), Cara

Therapeutics (CARA), as well as Zynerba Pharmaceuticals (ZYNE).

According to ArcView Market Research and also BDS Analytics, spending on legal marijuana is poised to grow 230% worldwide from $9.5 billion in 2017 to $31.3% billion in 2022, 33% of which is anticipated to go toward the clinical marijuana sector. Most of this number will be invested in the United States.

The range of items offered for recreational cannabis comes with a catch: significant taxes. Firms entailed in leisure cannabis items will certainly have to account for considerable governing fees from governments on their balance sheets.

DISTINGUISHING BETWEEN HEMP AS WELL AS CANNABIS

It has led to many rumours about what makes hemp various from cannabis. Whatever form *hemp plants are male as well as marijuana plants are female* to *marijuana is a medication and also the other is not* are incorrectly being preached as common knowledge to unknowing bystanders.

"Health Canada specifies hemp as products of Cannabis Sativa which consist of less than 0.3% THC, whereas US law defines hemp as all parts of any Cannabis Sativa plant having no psychedelic buildings, except defined exemptions."

According to several 1976 studies published by the International Association for Plant Taxonomy *"Cannabis Sativa, all hemp varieties and marijuana varieties, are of the same genus, Cannabis Sativa, as well as the same varieties. It is better to say that various varieties fell into other groups within the Cannabis Sativa varieties."*

Nonetheless, depending upon how the plant is expanded and also utilised will undoubtedly identify which term is proper. For example, the term marijuana (or cannabis) is used when defining a Cannabis Sativa plant that is reproduced for its potent, resinous glands (called trichomes). These trichomes include high amounts of tetrahydrocannabinol (THC), the cannabinoid most recognised for its psychedelic buildings.

Hemp, on the other hand, is made use of to explain a Cannabis Sativa plant which contains only trace quantities of THC. Hemp is a high-growing plant, commonly bred for industrial usages such as oils and topical lotions, along with fibre for apparel, building and construction, and also far more.

Only items made from industrial hemp (less than 0.3% THC) are lawful to offer, acquire, take in, and ship. This single factor (0.3%) is just how many people distinguish between what is categorised as hemp as well as what is identified as cannabis. This limit has caused mass controversy (for a good reason), which we will certainly dive into a little bit later on. But initially, allow's have a look at just how hemp is made use of all over the world.

Industrial hemp uses

From hemp apparel and also accessories to diets and hempseed oil cosmetics, the plant is seemingly found almost everywhere you look. Hemp can be made into wax, material, rope, towel paper and gas, among numerous various other points.

The entertainment cannabis market mostly makes use of THC (tetrahydrocannabinol), a psychedelic representative that is responsible for the high that comes from cigarette smoking marijuana, for its items. It has numerous applications across subjects, from marijuana-infused beer to coffee and cigarettes. Rather than having a clinical purpose, this sector markets the high that marijuana is known for and that numerous individuals look for.

According to the report launched by ArcView Market Research as well as BDS Analytics mentioned over, 67% of global marijuana spending is anticipated to happen in the entertainment market a massive draw for capitalists. However, the federal legalisation of recreational marijuana is vital before the marketplace can reach its true potential.

An additional alternative is to consider an exchange-traded fund (ETF), as limited as they are in the marketplace. These tools trade similar to stocks; however, pool with each other properties such as bonds, commodities, and products. The Alternative Harvest ETF includes firms such as GW Pharmaceuticals as well as Tilray as well as was trading at $33.23 as of 2019 May 28.

Hemp paper until the mid 19th century, hemp and flax were the two boss paper-making materials. In ancient times, a paper was refined from hemp cloth. Making use of hemp directly for the paper was taken into consideration also expensive, because of its absence of need at the time. Wood-based paper entered usage when mechanical as well as chemical pulping was established in the mid-1800s in Germany as well as England. Today, at the very least, 95% of paper is made from wood pulp. This makes little sense when taking into consideration hemp can easily create far more paper per acre than wood pulp options.

According to Hemp: A New Crop with New Uses for North America *the essential bast fibres in the bark are 5-40 mm long, as well as are integrated into fibre bundles which can be 1-5 m long (additional bast fibres are about 2 mm long). The woody core fibres are short-- about 0.55 mm-- as well as like wood fibres are sealed along with significant lignin. The core fibres are typically taken into consideration too short for high-grade paper applications (size of 3 mm is taken into consideration ideal), and excessive lignin is present."*

Hemp for paper

Because of its fibre size and also toughness, one of the factors hemp is so valuable is. These long bast fibres have been made use of to make paper almost for two millennia. Thomas Jefferson composed both the Declaration of Independence as well as the U.S. Constitution on hemp paper.

So, how does this all accumulate for investors? The basic structure for reviewing medical cannabis supplies stays similar to that for the pharmaceutical industry, which suggests financiers need to focus on the company's pipe of drugs as well as costs on the study. It is risk-free to presume that the payback for capitalists in this sector will undoubtedly be much longer as compared to leisure cannabis because research in marijuana is reasonably brand-new. For context, take into consideration that GW Pharmaceuticals spent nineteen years looking into cannabis chemicals before obtaining its first drug approval earlier this year.

The hemp paper procedure likewise makes use of much less power as well as fewer chemicals than tree paper handling and also doesn't produce the hazardous dioxins, chloroform, or anyone of the various other 2,000 chlorinated organic compounds that have been recognized as results of the wood paper process.

Only like clinical cannabis, there are supplies and also various other financial investments readily available in the leisure cannabis sector. The most famous company entailed in recreational marijuana play is Canadian player Canopy Growth (CGC).

What is hemp? Understanding the differences between hemp and cannabis

When attempting to fold your head over the differences between hemp as well as marijuana, it is essential, to begin with, this straightforward principle: Both hemp and marijuana inevitably come from the same plant merely different components. Whether you call something hemp or marijuana will undoubtedly rely on a selection of elements which we will check out in this publication. However, although the terms hemp and cannabis are frequently made use of reciprocally, they do have different undertones.

Uruguay, as well as Canada, are the only two countries that have legalised both entertainment and also medical marijuana for its citizens.

Entertainment marijuana stocks

Even though medical marijuana was legislated initially and also already has a semblance of distribution facilities in the form of medical dispensaries, entertainment cannabis satisfies a bigger audience and has a higher recall in public memory. This head start converts right into a potentially more significant market for this type of marijuana and is reflected in the rapid development stats for the business involved in this field.

Getting involved in the marketplace is as easy as any other industry. Investors might think about acquiring stock in business looking into or those that presently have clinical cannabis on the market, as stated above. Numerous are provided on stock exchanges like the Toronto Stock Exchange (TSX), while multiple is traded over the counter (OTC).

Additionally, oil stemmed from hemp seed has revealed a guarantee in treating eczema (persistent dry skin) in patients, although whole-plant cannabis oil has been verified to be a lot more reliable in handling a lot more severe skin problems, like skin cancer cells.

Hemp for food

Research studies have revealed consumption of raw hemp seeds can aid reduced blood pressure as well as cholesterol, increase weight loss, improve one's immune system, control blood sugar levels, and also reduce inflammation. This makes hemp seeds exceptionally healthy.

Hemp oil its raw kind, hemp has the secondhighest amount of protein of any food (soy being the greatest). Nonetheless, because the hemp seed's healthy protein a lot more carefully looks like the protein discovered in human blood, it is much easier to digest than soy protein. Hemp seeds can be consumed entire, pushed right into oil, or ground right into flour for baking.

In America, items originated from hemp seed, such as hemp seed spreads, hemp seed energy bars, hemp seed meal, as well as hemp oil-- are widely available in health food stores such as Whole Foods or Trader's supermarkets.

Hemp for health & body

Hemp seed oil is flawlessly suited for hair as well as skincare. Its dietary value, incorporated with its moisturising as well as renewing EFA's, makes it one of the very best vegetable body treatment structures. Hemp seed oil's EFA enhance consists of polyunsaturated fats, omega-3, omega-6, omega-9, linoleic acid, as well as gamma linoleic acids (GLA's). Although they are efficient in skin treatment upkeep, GLA's are rarely found in all-natural oils. Hemp is a superb source of GLA's.

Hemp for Fuel

Hemp seeds have supplied a combustible gas oil throughout social background. Necessarily, hemp can give two kinds of fuel:

1. Hemp biodiesel-- made from the oil of the (pressed) hemp seed.

2. Hemp ethanol/methanol-- made from the fermented stalk.

The principle of using oil derived from veggies as an engine gas is nothing brand-new. In 1895, Dr Rudolf Diesel developed the initial diesel motor to operate on vegetable oil-- peanut oil to be precise. You are producing hemp biodiesel when you push the hemp seeds and draw out the fat. Additionally, via processes such as gasification, hemp can be used to make both ethanols as well as methanol.

The controversy of classifying: hemp vs cannabis

A Canadian scientist created the worldwide interpretation of hemp (rather than marijuana) in 1971 that passes the name of Ernest Small Small's arbitrary 0.3% THC limitation has come to be typical around the globe as the main restriction for legal hemp, after he released an obscure, yet extremely significant book entitled The Species Problem in Cannabis. *"There is not any all-natural factor at which the cannabinoid material can be utilised to differentiate strains of hemp and also marijuana."*

There is a significant distinction between hemp seed oil, and also hemp/CBD remove. Products having hemp/CBD extract do have a wide range of cannabinoids, restricted to no THC. These kinds of products can be useful for increasing the high quality of one's life; many clients report that they have discovered relief for a broad range of disorders from hemp remove alone.

In this very same publication, Small talks about exactly how *"there is none all-natural factor at which the cannabinoid material can be made use of to differentiate strains of hemp as well as marijuana."* Despite this, Small remained to *"draw an approximate line on the continuum of marijuana kinds, and also determined that 0.3 per cent THC in a sifted set of marijuana blossoms was the distinction between hemp and cannabis."* As you can visualise, this has resulted in some dispute and also complication as to what makes up the distinction between hemp and even marijuana.

Hemp seed oil and hemp extract vs cannabis oil

Hemp seed oil is drawn out by pushing the seeds of the women's cannabis hemp plant. The hemp oil removed is healthy in regards to a dietary supplement; however, hemp seed oil lacks cannabinoids, which are the primary compounds located in the cannabis plant that can aid fight cancer. Hemp seed oil is discovered mainly in products in your regional supermarket and also generally includes two times the levels of omega-three found in olive oil with only fifty per cent of the complete calories.

Clients seeking to deal with even more severe illness as well as persistent diseases will undoubtedly wish to explore whole-plant marijuana oil therapies (i.e., Rick Simpson Oil). Products containing entire plant cannabis oil supply high doses of concentrated cannabinoids (e.g., THC, CBD, CBN, CBG, etc.), terpenes, as well as other substances from the plant that many clients, as well as caretakers, need to assist find relief from a wide range of condition

Furthermore, your location will undoubtedly identify your understanding of what constitutes hemp vs marijuana. For instance, Health Canada specifies hemp as items of Cannabis Sativa which have much less than 0.3 per cent THC, whereas U.S. regulation specifies hemp as all components of any Cannabis Sativa plant consisting of no psychoactive properties, besides defined exceptions.

A recent lawsuit between Hemp Industries Association v. DEA wrapped up *"the DEA can control foods containing natural THC if it is consisted of within marijuana, as well as can manage artificial THC of any kind. Yet they can not manage naturally-occurring THC not had within or stemmed from cannabis i.e., non-psychoactive hemp items because non-psychoactive hemp is not included in Schedule".*

HOW CANNABIS BENEFITS WOMEN'S GYNECOLOGICAL HEALTH

The ECS regulates these numerous features with substances called endocannabinoids, which bind to cannabinoid receptors in mind as well as throughout the worried peripheral system as well as the body's immune system. As variations happen and also a function becomes out of balance, the EC system reacts by manufacturing endocannabinoids as needed. Those endocannabinoids after that bind with cannabinoid receptors, triggering a series of chain reactions that bring features back to stabilise, so they run efficiently.

According to Forbes, the global cannabis sector is approximated to be worth $7.7 billion. It's forecasted to hit $31.4 billion by 2021.

The market is expanding partly since marijuana can be a functional type of medication. Several research studies have found that cannabis has the potential to assist with a range of medical problems, including anxiety, chronic pain, as well as epilepsy.

What this suggests for ladies' gynaecological health and wellness is that any reproductive problems they have that relate to a shortage in endocannabinoids may also be profited by marijuana usage and also the absorption of cannabinoids.

That's where the benefit of cannabis is available. Cannabis includes more than 100 plant-derived cannabinoids, called phytocannabinoids. Like endocannabinoids, these cannabis-derived cannabinoids can connect with the body's cannabinoid receptors. The cannabinoids derived from cannabis can serve to supplement the body's very own endocannabinoids, helping guarantee the ECS performs its law duties effectively.

Research studies have even revealed that this interaction, in between cannabis-derived cannabinoids and also the

ECS, can be valuable for conditions that have been linked to ECS dysregulation, including numerous sclerosis, Alzheimer's illness, as well as amyotrophic lateral sclerosis (ALS).

If hemp is legal in your state and also you're aiming to attempt it, but uncertain which pressures the most excellent fit your demands, we've obtained you covered. Have a look at our guide to marijuana strains listed below.

Newbie's guide to marijuana strains.

We might earn a small compensation if you purchase something via a link on this web page on how this works.

Cannabis usage gets on the rise in the United States. A 2018 research study clarifies that, while cannabis usage among teenagers has lowered, American grownups are significantly making use of marijuana on the everyday.

But, as any recreational or medical marijuana customer can tell you, not all marijuana is produced an equivalent. Different pressures of cannabis generate different effects, and also hence can be used for various reasons.

Marijuana evokes its effects on the body by engaging with the endocannabinoid system, or ECS. The ECS is a major self-regulatory network that is responsible for regulating a large variety of features, such as mood, metabolism, cravings, body immune system reaction, pain response, and also a lot more. The endocannabinoid system additionally plays an indispensable part in female reproductive processes.

Often, however, the ECS can come to be deficient in endocannabinoids. This can cause endocannabinoid system dysregulation, bring about inequality in the body and also eventually wellness issues.

According to Forbes, the global marijuana market is calculated to be worth $7.7 billion. It is expected to strike $31.4 billion by 2021.

A lot of market experts, however, are reevaluating the hybrid, Sativa and also indica groups. Sequel to Amos Elberg, head of information science at Confident Cannabis, these terms are essentially meaningless.

What this suggests for ladies' gynaecological wellness is that any reproductive problems they have that relate to a shortage in endocannabinoids might also be benefitted by marijuana use and the absorption of cannabinoids.

That is where the advantage of marijuana is available. Cannabis consists of greater than one hundred plant-derived cannabinoids, called phytocannabinoids. Like endocannabinoids, these cannabis-derived cannabinoids can communicate with the body's cannabinoid receptors. In essence, the cannabinoids derived from cannabis can offer to supplement the body's endocannabinoids, aiding make sure the ECS executes its policy obligations successfully.

Put, individuals shouldn't be distressed if a supposedly invigorating Sativa pressure has even more of a mellowing effect, or if an indica strain makes them feel extra bubbly as well as quick-tempered.

If you have reviewed a little regarding cannabis, or if you get in most dispensaries, you may see the words indica, Sativa, and also hybrid. Usually, most people divide cannabis right into these three categories.

However, as any medical or leisure cannabis user can inform you, not all marijuana is produced an equivalent. Different strains of marijuana produce different results, as well as this, can be made use of multiple factors.

Beyond Sativa, indica, and crossbreed, dispensaries might divide the types of marijuana they have into pressures. Strains are fundamentally different breeds of marijuana, and they are reproduced to have specific results on the individual.

Indica, that originates in the Hindu Kush mountains of India, is believed to have a soothing effect on the consumer.

Sativa has a more refreshing result, while crossbreed is a combination of both.

If cannabis is lawful in your state and you want to try it, yet unsure which pressures most exceptional fit your demands, we have got you covered. Take a look at our guide to cannabis pressures below.

The sector is growing in part since marijuana can be a versatile type of medication. A variety of study studies have discovered that cannabis has the possible to help with a variety of medical problems, consisting of stress and anxiety, chronic discomfort, as well as epilepsy.

And yet if the terms indica, Sativa, and hybrid are necessarily ineffective classifications, are strain names likewise meaningless?

Gold Acapulco

Invented from Acapulco, Mexico, Gold Acapulois a widely known and also hugely commended pressure of cannabis. It is noted for its euphoria-inducing, energising impacts. It is claimed to decrease exhaustion, anxiety, discomfort, and even nausea or vomiting.

White Widow

White Widow boosts your mood, offers you energy, as well as relaxes you at one time. It is said to help reduce discomfort and also stress, along with sensations of clinical depression. White Widow may assist you to remain invigorated and sharp if you are feeling worn down.

The strains should be extra or less regular if you purchase an item from a quality resource. Bear in mind, however, that every person acts in response in different ways to marijuana.

Super Silver Haze

An additional stimulating pressure, Super Silver Haze is said to produce feelings of euphoria, alleviates discomfort and queasiness, and also raises your mood. It makes it outstanding for stress alleviation.

TALK TO YOUR DOCTOR

If you are interested in trying marijuana, and also you are wanting to assist treat a clinical condition or currently taking any medicines, talk with your medical professional initially.

Different kinds of strains

According to user testimonials on Leafly, here is what people may anticipate from a few of the most popular cannabis pressures.

It is additionally worth researching the potential adverse results of the pressure. A lot of the more moderate demands, which you can locate below, checklist dry mouth, dry eyes, and dizziness as possible adverse effects. Marijuana additionally has the prospective to engage with medications you could be taking. Do not operate machinery when making use of marijuana.

Maui Wowie

Maui Wowie can help you feel extremely relaxed, yet energetic and creative. It lowers fatigue, too, making it excellent for days when you require to be effective.

There are, nonetheless, still consistencies amongst product sold under particular stress names, Elberg adds.

Bubba Kush

Bubba Kush is a relaxing, sleep-inducing pressure. It is ideal for aiding you battle insomnia and get some shut-eye. It additionally provides pain-reducing, stress-relieving results.

Not all seeds sold under the same name are genetically identical or possibly necessarily related. Some producers may select to develop a stress name basically as a branding exercise, or to recognise their product with an existing name because they believe the item matches characteristics the market anticipates from the product sold under that name Elberg describes.

Grandfather Purple

Grandfather Purple is an additional, very peaceful strain. It is often commended for its insomnia-fighting and also stress-reducing outcomes. Individuals also keep in mind that it can make you really feel ecstasy and also raise appetite, which is great if you're experiencing a lack of hunger.

Sour Diesel

A very stimulating, mood-lifting pressure, Sour Diesel is fantastic for offering you a ruptured of productive power. It likewise has notable destressing and also pain-relieving impacts.

LA Confidential

LA Confidential is an additional relaxing and also sleep-inducing pressure that is commonly made use of to soothe sleeplessness. It is likewise claimed to have visible anti-inflammatory and pain-reducing results, which makes it a preferred among individuals with chronic pain.

Northern Lights.

Northern Lights is one more relaxing, sleep-inducing stress. It is also understood for its mood-lifting results, and it can be utilised to relieve sleeplessness, clinical depression, pain, as well as stress and anxiety.

Fruity Pebbles

Fruity Pebbles OG, or FPOG, is related to generating ecstasy and relaxation, which could make it great for stress alleviation. It usually makes customers feel giggly, helps reduce nausea, and also raises appetite.

Blue Dream

Blue Dream is relaxing and soothing, however, it isn't a total sedative. When you can not manage to drop asleep, this makes it ideal for alleviating pain, pains, or inflammation. Plus, it is claimed to raise your mood as well as offer you a feeling of euphoria.

Accurately how to select a strain

The pressure you pick depends upon what effect you desire. As stated earlier, cannabis has a variety of clinical usages, yet some strains are better for certain conditions than others.

Golden Goat

Golden Goat is noteworthy for making customers feel creative and also euphoric. It is additionally excellent for lowering exhaustion and stress and anxiety while raising your mood. Not specifically, says Elberg.

Purple Kush

Purple Kush is excellent for inducing a state of bliss to make sure that you feel unwinded, happy, as well as tired. It is usually used for minimising pain and also muscle spasms. Its sedating impacts means it can be utilised to reduce sleep problems.

Covering Kush

Originating from the Hindu Kush hills near the Afghanistan-Pakistan boundary, Afghan Kush is incredibly relaxing and also sleep-inducing. This, too, can assist you to feel hungry if you are experiencing an absence of cravings, and also can eliminate pain.

Essential items

On the off chance that marijuana is legitimate in your state and also you're interested in attempting or perhaps growing various sorts of cannabis pressures, there are a variety of items that can make your life a little much more comfortable.

Pineapple Express

Put on the map by the 2008 eponymous film, Pineapple Express has a pineapple-like fragrance. It is kicking back and also a state of mind lifting, however, it is additionally said to give you an energetic buzz. This is the sort of pressure that could be excellent for performance.

Harvest Starter Kit

If you want to begin expanding your marijuana, this practical starter kit includes everything you need to harvest it. Unfortunately, it only checks liquids, not dried natural herb.

Helpful items

In the event that cannabis is lawful in your state and also you are interested in attempting-- and even growing various sorts of marijuana stress, several products can make your life a little much more comfortable.

One of the most frequently asked questions we obtain from clients is: *"What is the appropriate everyday dosage of CBD for me?"* If you do a Google search on CBD dose, you will undoubtedly find various dimensions as well as approximate dosages for different products. The fact is, this is a complicated concern to answer.

There are several factors that require to be thought about when locating the perfect dose of CBD for you. Several of the variables that play a vital part in your experience making use of CBD are:

The grow set includes a trimming tray, a microscope for analysing the buds to determine whether they're all set for harvest, three sorts of pruning shears, a sanitising spray for your tools, a drying out shelf, and also gloves.

Keep in mind: Even if cannabis is legal in your state, it continues to be unlawful under federal regulation

- Rest problems such as insomnia.
- Migraine headaches and also other kinds of headaches.
- Mood swings.
- Nausea or vomiting and menopausal symptoms.
- PTSD Posttraumatic Stress Disorder.
- Tension as well as restlessness.
- Metabolic disorders.
- For the microdose, we suggest our 500mg CBD oil. One decrease in 500mg oil includes 2 mg of CBD.

Magical Butter Kit

Cannabutter or cannabis-infused butter is the basis of numerous edibles. Unfortunately, making cannabutter can be a labour-intensive and lengthy procedure.

Leinow & Birnbaum suggest that to begin with, a microdose, typical dosage and even microdose, depending upon the sort of signs and symptoms.

If you have picked among the dosage tables (see below), search for your body weight in the left column. Make use of the approximate value as an overview if it lies in between the amounts are shown.

Beginning at the lowest daily dose under Step 1. This is your starting dosage. Maintain it for one week.

Listen to your body and also take notes if required. If essential, you can, after that increase the dose to the following action, maintain it for one week and more. The declines do not need to be taken at one time. For more significant amounts, it is a good idea to divide the drops right into lunchtime, evening and also early morning.

If you discover any unfavorable effects, minimise the dosage. It is not an inquiry of increasing the dosage steadily, but of finding the perfect dosage. Because of the two-phase impact, both an as well low and a too high dose are much less reliable.

When you have discovered a dose that you feel comfortable with, maintain it. This will be your target dosage from now on.

The numbers represent the variety of decreases and also the focus of CBD oil. Instance: 6 x 5 stands for six drops of 500mg CBD oil. CBD oil with various focus can be replaced (Example: Four declines of 1500mg CBD oil correspond to twelve declines of 500mg CBD oil).

CBD is an acronym for Cannabidiol. A substance component discovered in hemp and marijuana that does not have the addictive and also invigorating effects related to other marijuana compounds such as Tetrahydrocannabinol (THC). As a result of this, it is legal, marketed and made use of in lots of countries around the world.

Palm Mincer

Grinding up marijuana can be time-consuming so that the Palm Mincer can be fairly valuable. It fits completely into your hand, as well as it can be made use of to cut up marijuana quickly and also effectively. What's more, it is dishwasher secure, so it's simple to clean off the sticky cannabis resin. You can buy it below.

- Your clinical condition or issue.
- Exactly how extreme your issue is.
- Metabolism.
- Exactly how you react to CBD.
- Body Weight.
- Level of sensitivity to cannabis.
- Your body chemistry (this consists of any other medicines you might be taking).

So, How Much CBD Should You Take?

Based upon the standard in the guide, we suggest the step-up method were you gradually raise the dose till the most desired results are reached. The term used in the guide is *Titration*. This is a term borrowed from chemistry that suggests taking small actions in time to permit adjustment gradually. By using this technique, you are tailoring the quantity of oil to fit your requirements. Every person is different, as well as every person's response to CBD is different.

TCheck Dosage Checker

The *Check Dosage Checker* checks the strength of cannabis-infused fluids-- like alcohol-based casts. It can also test cannabis-infused olive oil, ghee (explained margarine), and coconut spread, which will certainly help you figure out just how reliable your edibles are before you delight.

What's the Right Dose of CBD?

CBD is an all-natural plant substance, consequently, according to the World's Health Organization (WHO) its risk-free to eat as long as it is tidy as well as has no contaminants. We have placed with each other this basic dosage overview which adheres to the dose overview led to out in a publication labelled *CBD: A Patient's Guide To Medical* Cannabis by Leonard Leinow and Juliana Birnbaum. They are experts in CBD leaders in this facet of the industry.

MicroDose

0.5 mg to 20mg of CBD per dose each day (CBD/dose/day) is a microdose recommended for the list below conditions:

EXPANDING LAWS

Regulation around growing cannabis varies from one state to another. Before you decide to cultivate, ensure you have done your research.

Volcano Vaporizer

Some individuals could like breathing in cannabis over smoking it via a pipeline, bong, or joint. This desktop vaporiser warms up marijuana and also expels the vapour into a balloon. The individual then breathes in the air from the aircraft.

This publication *Cannabis Cookbook* is an excellent source for those who have not yet considered CBD and also its medical homes. The book contains information concerning the advantages of food preparation with marijuana, its background, usage, dosage, researches on its use in a selection of diseases, and a lot more.

This butter package, however, makes it easy to instil natural herbs into butter. It has its own home heating system as well as a thermostat, which ensures that the product as well as butter are at an excellent temperature level throughout the procedure.

Fruity Pebbly

Fruity Pebbles OG, or FPOG, is related to causing ecstasy and furthermore unwinding, which can make it spectacular for uneasiness alleviation. It frequently makes users feel giggly, helps reduce queasiness, as well as enhances hunger.

The vaporizer can be made use of with dried natural herbs or fluid concentrates, and can be purchased below.

CANNABIS DOSING GUIDE

CBD DOSAGE: HOW MUCH CBD SHOULD I TAKE

Cancer, epilepsy, liver illness.

For a macrodose, we recommend our 30%, 40% or 50% CBD paste. For the 1500mg oil: 3 declines 3 times per day = 54mg of CBD.

CBD.

For the 2500mg oil: 3 decreases 3 times each day = 60mg of CBD. Chart Standard dosage: Number of decreases x CBD oil concentration.

Macro (Or Therapeutic) Dose

Macro dosages are at the wide variety between 50mg-800mg of CBD/dose/day. This dose is frequently made use of for:

Chart Micro dosage: Number of drops x CBD oil focus

Standard Dose

10mg to 100mg of CBD/dose/day. Common doses are made use of for the list below conditions:

- Persistent pain
- Inflammations
- Autoimmune illness
- Lyme condition
- Anxiousness condition
- Clinical depressions
- Fibromyalgia
- Several sclerosis
- Autism
- Crohn's illness and also IBS (irritable digestive tract disorder).
- Rheumatoid joint inflammation.

For a conventional dose, we advise our 1500mg or 2500mg CBD oil. One decrease of the 1500mg CBD oil contains 6mg of CBD, and also one reduction of the 2500mg oil includes 6,7 mg of CBD.

30% paste: 1 millilitre contains 300mg of CBD.

40% paste: 1 milliliter contains 400mg of CBD.

50% paste: 1 milliliter consists of 500mg of CBD.

Determining effectiveness is one of the toughest parts of making edibles because most individuals do not know the cannabinoid content of their beginning product. Unless you approach a testing office, knowing the cannabinoid composition of your starting herb or concentrate is much easier said than done.

Despite the fact that this may sound confusing, my companion Jeff the four-hundred-twenty chefs has assembled a user-accommodating number cruncher to help you to recognize how a lot of cannabis items and furthermore oil/spread must be utilized for any recipe. It will likewise break down the mg of THC or CBD in each offering dimension.

The bright side is, you can use ordinary THC (or CBD) portions of the beginning material to aid ballpark the strength degree of your edibles. We must emphasise is that edibles made from 7g of top-shelf, California sun-grown OG Kush flowers are mosting likely to be dramatically stronger than edibles made from 7g of artificially grown trim.

This data pertains to THC-rich pressures (i.e. the stuff that is intended to obtain you high, a lot of street weed) instead of clinically oriented high-CBD strains, which typically have reduced degrees of THC, or organic hemp flour, which contains less than 0.3% THC according to government guidelines. When it comes to the bud itself, lawful states like Colorado will certainly balance even more like 18% THC, whereas non-legal countries could be closer to 10% THC. Chart Macro dose: Number of declines x CBD oil concentration.

General Dosage Guidelines

When it comes to CBD dose, it is essential to bear in mind that there is not a one size fits all. The dosage quantity varies from specific to private, relying on several factors mentioned earlier. It is suggested to consult your healthcare company for advice on how much CBD you must take.

Do not also take much CBD. It is vital to keep in mind that in cannabis treatment frequently times "much less is more" If you are not obtaining the wanted outcomes from a higher dosage than you need to take into consideration lowering your dose instead of boosting it.

Be aware of possible side results and also medicine interactions if you are currently taking some various other prescription drugs. You need to review this with your healthcare carrier.

Regularly talk to a medical care expert

For a medical condition, always consult with a healthcare expert before consuming CBD. Any details contained in or made readily available through any advertising materials are not meant to be used as, or be a replacement for, medical care recommendations or details from qualified healthcare specialists.

The next action is to figure out how many servings the recipe makes: does it make twelve or twenty-four cookies? Increase the variety of portions in the method by the wanted THC content in each meal; this will undoubtedly generate the total amount of THC in mg required to attain your preferred potency degree.

Below you will discover a chart that explains typical results felt at different ingested dosages. Nonetheless, there are variables to think about when choosing the right dosage for you, which you can read more regarding below.

Required aid establishing the strength of your cannabis? Besides aesthetic examination, you can do a quick smoke test and place it amongst the other strains you have smoked. The following table reveals the series of average THC per cent by weight in each sort of beginning material:

We like the organic, non-GMO, federally lawful hemp flower strains developed by Canna Comforts. Each varietal looks, smells, preferences, as well as smokes just like the top-shelf cannabis pressure that motivated it, producing a superior medical cigarette smoking or vaping experience as well as delicious whole-plant concentrates. As their items are separately tested for effectiveness, high quality, as well as pureness, calculating dosage is easier with hemp blossom than with standard cannabis.

Edible types of marijuana, consisting of food tablets, pills, and also items, can generate efficient, lasting, and also risk-free impacts. These types of cannabis are additionally the most likely to produce undesirable effects as well as overdose signs and symptoms, which can be undesirable. The distinction is, naturally, the dose.

If you are making use of already-infused coconut oil and also it's reliable, you can weaken it with added coconut oil to decrease its focus. Then again, if it is excessively feeble, you can re-infuse or include a small measure of exceptionally focused cannabis coconut oil to the thin-set. It may take several batches before you attain your highest dosage, yet it will without a doubt get substantially more agreeable and progressively exact each time.

While you might understand you can make use of CBD oils to include a healing strike to your food, did you know you can additionally use natural hemp flower to develop full-spectrum, food-safe, custom CBD essences at home?

The easiest way to determine the amount of marijuana beginning material needed is to back right into the number based on what you think about to be an individual dose of THC. For some individuals, this is 5mg of THC, and for others, it is in extra of 100mg. For more on how to select the right dosage for you, have a look at our detailed consumption overview.

HEMP SEEDS FOR WEIGHT LOSS

Losing those extra pounds is going to drive you insane. In addition to the exercise, walk as well as keeping an eye on your carbs; you have to ensure that you do not starve your body from fatty acids and vital, healthy proteins.

Do you know what you require? An ingredient that is high in healthy protein and also short on carbs.

Hailed as a SuperFood by many wellness experts, hemp seeds are perfect for shedding weight. They have a plethora of benefits with one of the ideal mix of protein, omega-three fatty acid, iron, fibre, magnesium and also zinc.

HEMP HEARTS VS HEMP SEEDS

Individuals typically choose hemp hearts over hemp seeds. I mean necessarily both the seeds are very same types that are Hemp.

Cookies, delicious chocolates, as well as other food items can likewise be made use of if they are purposefully held in the mouth for 1-3 minutes before ingesting. Oils and tinctures are typically the simplest to make use of for precise application and also progressively increasing the dose to find what jobs best for you.

I encourage those brand-new to cannabis edibles to wait for two hours before taking an extra dosage of marijuana. The most typical blunder in marijuana dosing occurs when an individual doesn't feel any result from an edible after one hour as well as decides to take an additional dose; 2 hours later, the individual experiences the undesirable effects of an overdose. Application Recommendations for Consumers New to Cannabis Edibles

Beginning dose: 1-2.5 mg of THC (plus CBD if available/desired).

If you are uncertain if a particular dosage of cannabis is influencing you, I suggest finding out Healer's *Inner Inventory*, a quick as well as simple self-awareness tool that can be utilised to establish if you are feeling the effects of a specific dosage of marijuana.

More tips for consuming infused edibles.

If you do not feel any effects from an edible after one hour, attempt consuming a snack like an organic apple to activate the food digestion and also absorption in your intestine.

Some individuals that are brand-new to marijuana require two-three dosages before they feel anything, so it is commonly best to attempt the very same low dosage three times with eight to twenty-four hours between trials before raising the dose.

I have rarely satisfied patients who appear incapable of absorbing any substantial amount of THC with the intestine. In these individuals, absorption using the dental capillary or the lungs is the best alternative.

Tips for relieving an edibles-induced overdose

A calm, secure atmosphere and gentle reassurance that everything will be fine is the primary therapy.

Remain moisturised.

A large 50-200mg dose of CBD (without considerable amounts of THC) can function as a partial antidote. Lemon oil, discovered primarily in the rind and also in lower quantities in the juice, has likewise been made use of historically for this objective. Grate a tbsp of lemon enthusiasm and also chew it up before ingesting.

The majority of people do not need emergency medical care unless they have pre-existing heart disease or various other significant clinical problems. For ongoing vomiting and looseness of the bowels, intravenous rehydration might be required.

The right dose varies between individuals

Everyone has a distinct internal physiologic atmosphere and can, therefore, experience different outcomes with various medicines. Someone's reaction to a dose of edible marijuana can differ dramatically from the next, even more so than other drugs or herbs. Why? Several aspects are included, including a previous background of cannabis use, intestinal variables, as well as the function/sensitivity of one's endocannabinoid system. Approximately 3% of my patient's location ultra-sensitive to THC and also do well with very reduced dosages (e.g. 1mg).

Understand CBD as well as THC Contents

Adding CBD to THC can improve the clinical benefits, such as pain or stress and anxiety alleviation while reducing the unfavourable results, such as problems and also raised the heart rate. CBD partly obstructs the intoxicating effects of THC, so customers that wish to experience the medical benefits of marijuana without as much disability can best accomplish this with products that contain both CBD and THC. Customers must understand the content of each of these elements, and also the proportion of CBD to THC.

Below is a shocker: much fussed and also excited chia or flex seeds are dismissed by Hemp seeds when it pertains to offering a total package of nutrients.

The particular proportion of healthy protein, omega three fatty acids, iron, Magnesium is what makes it a powerhouse of nutrition.

Hemp seeds: nature's superfood

The long listing of advantages is what makes hemp seeds Superfood. Hemp seeds come from Cannabis Sativa plant, likewise called commercial hemp. Unlike cannabis, industrial hemp consists of non-existent THC traces that won't obtain you high. Yes, you listened to that right-

This is among the reasons that hemp seeds are expanding in appeal everyday.

Extreme doses of these products can still produce timeless marijuana overdose sAs the CBD: THC proportion rises, the probability of undesirable envigorating effects reduces, and the high quality of the medical impacts will certainly also alter. A person who feels impaired after taking 5mg of THC will likely feel less or no problems when taking 20mg of CBD + 5mg of THC.

Just how exactly hemp seeds support weight loss?

1) Rich in omega-3 fatty acids.

Hemp seeds are abundant in omega three and also six fatty acids in the best proportion (1:3) according to the nutritional needs of a body. The majority of Americans have deprived of omega-three fatty acids since our food includes omega-6 in excellent quality. This inequality per centage is the root cause of inflammation, numerous joint and muscle mass troubles, and heart diseases.

Since it has a light nutty flavour and a soft structure that will enhance any dish, you can quickly induce hemp hearts in your day-to-day eatables.

So, if you intend to consist of fibre-rich food in your everyday diet, then you will indeed not find anything better after that whole hemp seeds. Your just other option for such an abundant resource of fibre is sand, but we are no worms, bear in mind?

Well, undoubtedly, the difference below is between the outside as well as the structure. The hemp hearts are likewise known as hulled/shelled hemp seed because the crunchy external hull is eliminated in hemp hearts. You get a soft chewy as well as nutty inner only, and that is why it is mostly favoured.

Hull of the hemp seeds can aid with the cleansing of your intestinal tract and also clean up your colon.

Whole hemp seeds have their hard, crispy outside shell undamaged. If you like chewing on treats, hemp seeds are a great option.

Because of their hard, crunchy exterior, many people are often reluctant to add them to their recipes.

It is notable to discuss, that whole hemp seeds are a great resource of fibre and minerals. Indeed, when you get rid of the hull, a different source of fibre is being discarded and also keep in mind, this sort of grain is non-existent in today's diet plan.

Currently, How Exactly Omega-3 fatty acids can Aid in weight loss? Omega-3 fats are practical for the increase in metabolism, so the more food id burned by your body, the even more weight you lose. It is basic.

Also, the anti-inflammatory homes of hemp seeds aid increase your physical performance while exercising, hence helping you to lose more weight properly.

When you have your omega-3 and omega-6 fatty acids in ideal proportion, you will undoubtedly observe a couple of yearnings, as well as your hunger, will be complete. Talking from individual experience, Getting rids of desires is a practical action to your lighter self.

2) Loaded with complete protein

Hemp seeds are nature's rarest superfood filled with a total healthy protein with all twenty amino-acids and also nine essential amino acids. The healthy protein assists the weight-loss trip by keeping your blood sugar level in check and also your power level steady sufficient, so you do not crave for high-calorie, fattening food.

For muscle growth and also recuperation, amino acids are quite essential. Hemp seeds consist of one of the most vital L Arginine amino acids, which becomes nitric oxide in your body that aids the blood vessel loosen up, which consequently enhances up the body's blood circulation.

A 3 tablespoon serving of hemp seeds will undoubtedly provide you with 10gms of healthy protein and add some amount of iron, zinc, as well as magnesium.

3) Great source of fiber

Whole hemp seeds contain a significant quantity of fibre, both insoluble and soluble. Keep in mind; hemp hearts are deprived of this fantastic fibre resource and a lot of the trace elements.

Food with high fibre features several advantages-- it helps do away with toxic substances, cleanse your colon, and keep your intestine health on point.

Researches recommend that reduced sugar, as well as high fibre ratio, will undoubtedly stop your body from blood sugar level spikes so you will not hunger for pleasant food- a supreme weight gain perpetrator.

And when we speak about weight reduction, a study by the University of Massachusetts suggests that a high fibre diet can help with the weight decrease.

4) Contains GLA that helps in weight loss

Hemp seeds or hemp oil consists of a high amount of GLA (gamma-linoleic acid). According to the University of California research study, GLA aids in minimising weight as well as especially avoid weight gain that is a typical disadvantage after significant weight-loss.

Right here's how:

Hemp seeds have an unsaturated fatty acid account that has "great" fat essential to burn the "bad" fat.

GLA improves your metabolism and also provokes the adipose tissue (brownish fat) to melt calories to give you power. In case you are overweight, brownish fat is much less most likely to be active. So GLA triggers this brownish fat, and also; as a result, your body will burn white fat that is a frequently noticeable indication of obesity.

Adding hemp seeds to your diet will certainly make sure that you do not gain back those added pounds that you have worked so hard to lose.

Also, GLA abundant food help suppress your cravings as it elevates the serotonin levels in your body. Less hunger = much less consuming and boom- you lose weight!

Primarily, GLA is a fat discovered in omega six that is not just essential for hormonal agents health, managing swelling, and also hypertension, however likewise aids in weight management.

In this research, the researcher offered one team of previously overweight individuals evening primrose oil as well as another group of olive oil for one year. It was then observed that those taking GLA supplements had acquired less weight compared to those that have not.

5) Stamps out the food craving

The ever before first hemp seeds are addicting as well as delicious so you can bite on them whenever you long for some treats. The body does not easily digest the insoluble fibre, and so you feel satiated for a more extended period.

When your body is nourished, you are really feeling stimulated, and also your digestive tract health depends on the mark; you won't think about food for hours. Your brain is carrying out proficiently, thanks to omega-three fats.

Full nutritional value of hemp seeds

One serving of hemp seeds (3 tbsp.) consists of:

the mix of protein, healthy and balanced fat, as well as fibre, will undoubtedly maintain your body along with your mind in an ethical and stable form, and therefore dropping weight will come to be much easier for you.

High fatty acids and total protein account- both are gradually digesting active ingredients so your power level will certainly be up for many hours as well as you will not have the urge to have unhealthy food.

3000 mg omega-3 and omega-6 fatty acid in a perfect ratio of 1:3.

10 mg full protein that has all the nine essential amino acids, iron, Mmagnesium, and also phosphorus.

One such inspirational number is MIKE FATA, founder of Manitoba Harvest Hemp seeds Company Canada. Mike came to be a *ganjapreneur* because of a life-altering event in 1994 when he was eighteen as well as evaluated over three-hundred extra pounds. He tried magic diet regimens and deprived his body of fats, yet that made him also sicker.

Best ways to lose weight with cannabis seeds.

Hemp seeds are addictively tasty as well as such a flexible food that can perfectly blend right into any dish and also not just improves the preference yet likewise aid you to lose weight while giving all the crucial nutrients.

This life-altering journey motivated mike to launch an organisation to encourage individuals to select a healthy way of living and healthy food. Hence he started Manitoba Harvest hemp seeds Company in 1998.

Hemp seeds are the only plant-based healthy protein that contains all the amino acids, as well as it is digested much more comfortable than animal healthy protein such as eggs, meat, milk, and also cheese.

Up until someday, he was introduced to hemp seeds a fantastic source of fats and also healthy proteins- by a friend. He started looking into nutrition as well as came to know that our body requires some necessary fats.

By frequently exercising as well as including hemp seeds in his diet regimen- Mark lost regarding 1one-hundred pounds, and his weight came down to two-hundred extra pounds.

Individuals Who Lost Weight By Using Hemp Seeds. All the details over are based on research and many individuals have dropped weight significantly by the assistance of hemp seeds. Mark is a big sponsor of hemp food and nourishment as well as has appeared on TELEVISION, radio as well as paper since.

Is not that great?

Have a look at some of the fun as well as unique ways to integrate hemp seed in your daily diet.

Hemp hearts are a terrific way to begin your early morning. They have a luscious appearance which is optimal for smoothies. You can mix them in with berries, bananas or any other fruits for your morning or post-workout shakes.

Add some added problem to your salad by spraying hemp seeds over it. You can also utilise hemp oil as your salad dressing. Hemp oil is short on calories and also carbohydrates compared to olive oil, and the benefit is that it tastes terrific as well.

Hemp milk preferences a lot better than soy milk as well as is an all-natural resource of calcium. Lactose intolerant people can currently make their non-dairy hemp milk as well as trust me it is way much more comfortable than it sounds. Assimilate a mug of hemp seeds and three to four cups of water together. You can likewise include salt for other ting and if you like the flavour, assimilate any fruit. Refrigerate and also stress the mixture. So, your very own organic, as well as healthiest hemp milk, prepares.

When it comes to hemp hearts, there are a lot of choices. You can blend them into your healthy protein and granola bars; you can make cookies or spray them in addition to your chicken bread. Undoubtedly, you are going to be shocked at how these tiny grains, along with a lot of recipes, can assimilate.

Final Thoughts

Making hemp seeds apart of your daily food intake will certainly profit you in a lot of incredible methods. You will not only drop weight quickly, yet your mind, heart, as well as total body wellness, will enhance, as well as you will undoubtedly start feeling invigorated. This superfood is instilled with the unique nutritional profile that is sorely missing out on in the majority of modern-day food options.

SOME BENEFITS OF HEMP SEEDS

So no, the hemp seeds in your brain won't make you make fun of Pineapple Express, yet they could help you take pleasure in a much healthier life in the adhering to ways.

To reap the benefits, Shapiro recommends including one everyday tablespoon of hempseed-- also called hemp hearts-- to your diet plan in a variety of means. Mix them into your shake or bowl of oatmeal for the morning meal.

As well as at dinner or lunch, spray them in addition to your salad, grain bowl, or a plate of pasta.

hemp is now a bonafide superfood: *"Hemp is super-nutritious as well as although little, quite mighty"* said Amy Shapiro, R.D., founder of Real Nutrition.

Indeed, hemp does come from the very same family of plants like cannabis. But no, it will not get you high-- there's a distinctive difference between psychedelic and also non-psychoactive kinds of hemp, according to the journal Nutrition as well as Metabolism. Hemp seeds have less than 0.3% tetrahydrocannabinol (THC) which is incredibly minimal.

You can also attempt hemp milk a non-dairy choice made from mixing hemp hearts with water. Hemp butter-- ground-up hemp hearts-- makes a healthy peanut butter alternative.

"There are truly no negative side effects [to consuming hemp] except if you take blood coagulants, you should boost your hemp intake gradually as it may trigger bleeding threats" said Shapiro.

1. Hemp seeds can help develop muscle mass.

Miss the healthy protein powders and also add a dose of protein-rich hemp to your smoothie to change things up. Shapiro says that unlike most plant-based healthy protein sources, hemp seeds have all the essential amino acids, making it a complete healthy protein

2. They can boost power

Hemp seeds contain a small number of intricate carbs (regarding a gram per tbsp), which launches sugar gradually right into the bloodstream, according to The American Heart Association, and also protects against that feared power spike and even subsequent collision.

3. They may assist you to slim down

Fat burning occurs when you expend more calories than you take in, so hemp seeds will not singlehandedly help you drop extra pounds. Yet they could help *"if it changes fattier and also richer sorts of proteins in the diet"* such as red meat or whole-fat dairy, said Shapiro.

She adds that eating it in various other forms might additionally aid with weight loss. For instance, hemp milk has fewer carbs and sugars than regular dairy products milk, and hemp healthy protein powder is an excellent enhancement to smoothies to assist in regulating cravings.

4. Hemp seeds might maintain you from getting hangry

According to Shapiro, hemp seeds are packed with fibre, which is excellent for keeping you good and full for hours. So including hemp powder, hearts, or milk to your a.m. meal might be the secret to keeping that mid-morning wall mount away. Be sure to consume alcohol a lot of water to help maintain that fibre from hanging around in your GI tract.

5. They will aid you rest

Hemp is high in magnesium, which is a mineral that usually relaxes the body and kicks back muscle mass, claimed Shapiro. To promote high-quality sleep, she suggests eating a serving a couple of hrs before bed.

6. They can help fix anaemia

Shapiro said that due to its high iron web content, consuming hemp seeds is a fantastic way to combat or prevent the problem.

7. Hemp seeds might protect your ticker

Eating hemp seeds *"helps protect against cardiovascular disease, maintain arteries open and also decrease blood pressure"* said Shapiro, thanks to enough amount of omega-3 and omega-6 fatty acids. The seeds likewise include high quantities of arginine, which becomes nitric oxide in the body which is essential for optimum heart wellness.

8. They might reduce PMS signs

The excellent news: All those crucial fatty acids (EFA) in hemp seeds may assist all your PMS issues. FYI: You can get an equal amount of EFAs in a single offering of hemp oil or hemp seeds.

Primarily, people consume CBD, infused foodstuff to get remedy for discomfort and swelling. Research studies claim that CBD can minimise pain as well as supply remedy for signs of chronic discomfort. Unsurprisingly, CBD can be included in brownies similar to THC marijuana can be added. That way, it ends up being enjoyable as well as lovable to contain CBD to one's diet plan while appreciating your much-loved snack.

A lot of us like brownies right from our childhood years. Remarkably, brownie dishes developed a lot with fascinating and adorable combinations. Nevertheless, would you even think of consuming a chocolate brownie when you remain in intolerable and also exceptionally unpleasant pain

CBD is formulated from the marijuana plant, and also it is vegan. Nevertheless, CBD individuals are not limited to vegans or non-vegans. CBD brownies can be fit for human consumption with or without eggs. For the benefit of all, we will go over the preparation approaches for both vegans and also non-vegans.

Unlike THC brownies, CBD brownies are non-psychoactive as well as secure to eat by everyone. Better, self-cooked brownies tend to be hygienic and also more delicious than the ones you purchase from the retailers. Equally, consisting of CBD to the brownie makes it less complicated to make children take pleasure in a nutrition-rich diet.

Discover How To Make CBD Brownies Using CBD Oil.

CBD brownie for Vegans and also Non-Vegans

Non-Vegan CBD brownie

Ingredients

- 1/2 mug Flour
- 1 cup Sugar
- One mug of sunflower oil

- 1/3 cup Cocoa powder
- 1/2 teaspoon cooking powder
- 1/4 tsp salt
- One egg
- CBD oil
- Vanilla remove

Directions

Step 1:

The stove is to be preheated to 180 °. Now, blend the sunflower oil and also sugar in a dish until it gets combined thoroughly. Once it gets combined, include vanilla extract as well as CBD as required. Plus, add the eggs as well as stir the mix till it mixes well.

Step 2:

Individually, take a dish as well as include salt, flour, baking powder, and cacao powder. Include the damp mixture which you prepared in step 1 to the plate and also stir it well to blend it. Now you obtained the ideal brownie mix ready to frying pan.

Step 3:

Pour the mix right into a well-greased pan and cook till the sides of the brownie obtain separated from the frying pan. Place the prepared brownie on a plate and permit it to cool. Cut it right into pieces and also appreciate the brownies.

Except for the eggs, everything else remains the same to prepare a vegan CBD brownie. Ahead, you will undoubtedly be including sunflower oil, almond oil, and also apple sauce in the Vegan CBD brownie recipe.

Ingredients

- 3 cups of sugar
- 2 cups apple sauce
- 2 cups of cocoa powder
- Four mugs flour
- 1 1/2 tsp salt
- 1 cup almond milk
- One tablespoon vanilla essence
- 1 1/2 mugs sunflower oil
- CBD oil
- 1 tbsp cooking powder

Step 1:

Establish the preheat to 160 ° in the stove. Prepare the dry mix with chocolate powder, sugar, flour, and also salt by blending it well in a bowl. Guarantee it obtains blended well to avoid irregular or harsh surfaces on the brownie.

Step 2:

Prepare the damp-mix by adding sunflower oil, almond milk, apple sauce, CBD oil and also vanilla remove. Mix it well to blend it well.

Step 3:

Currently, put the wet mix in the bowl which contains the dry mix prepared symphonious 1. Mix whatever utilising a whisk, so that you get a smooth as well as best brownie mix.

Step 4:

Oil the pan and put the brownie mix to cook it till the sides get separated from the frying pan. Make slices and delight in the ideal vegan CBD brownie.

CBD brownies with vaped buds

Other than, at the last step, you should melt the chocolate and pour it on the prepared CBD brownie. On the top, sprinkle the vaped CBD buds on the dissolved chocolate. Virtually, including the vaped CBD buds to the brownies is the most natural preparation approach. Right from preparing the wet mix till cooking the brownies whatever is the same as the vegan CBD brownie.

CBD brownies with Cannabis butter

I hope you all know what is cannabis butter. To put it merely, exceptional CBD stress is added to the butter. In this way, cannabidiol obtains turned on. Before the chocolate is included in the brownie mix, cannabis butter has to be thawed and blended with the chocolate. By doing this, CBD obtains added to the recipe without disrupting the actual preference as well as the flavour of the brownie.

Wrap:

CBD brownies are an excellent way to include CBD in your diet. Having claimed that, preparing it on your own makes it genuine and also more delicious. Also, if you learn to cook CBD infused foods on your own, then you can tailor the flavour based on your requirements. Exactly, making brownies with proper CBD dosage is essential to stay clear of any undesirable adverse effects. Besides, it aids in stopping the preference of CBD from disturbing the real taste of the brownie.

Thai High

Do you like cannabis and do you love mixed drinks? What could be much better than bringing the two with each other?

Thai High

- 1 1/2 oz Bacardi light rum
- 1/2 oz Capitol Hill Heat habanero-smoke cannabis syrup (approx. 10 mg THC)
- 1/2 oz fresh-squeezed lime juice.
- 2 oz pineapple juice

Thai basil to garnish

Incorporate rum, lime, pineapple and syrup juice, and shake well with ice up until altogether chilled. Twofold strain into a collins glass over fresh ice, top with soda water, stir and furthermore garnish with a sprig of Thai basil (for perfect results, yet the sprig lightly on the palm of your hand to open up its fragrances).

- 2 oz bourbon.
- 1/2 oz Ginger Grass ginger cannabis syrup (approx. 10mg THC) *.
- 1/2 oz fresh-squeezed lemon juice.
- 1/2 oz honey syrup.
- Four pieces of fresh peeled ginger.
- Lemon peel off to garnish.

Smoke with Spices.

Muddle ginger slices in a shaker, then add ice as well as continuing to be ingredients and also shake well till thoroughly chilled. Stress into a cooled coupe glass and also garnish with a lemon spin.

- 1 1/2 oz tequila reposado.
- 3/4 oz Cointreau.
- 1 oz Capitol Hill Heat habanero-smoke marijuana syrup (approx. 20mg THC)
- 1 oz fresh-squeezed lime juice.
- 1 oz fresh-squeezed lemon juice.
- One dashboard Tabasco (optional).

Lime wedge to prepare

Include all ingredients to a shaker with ice and also shake until thoroughly chilled. Pressure into a rocks glass with fresh ice as well as serve.

- 1 1/2 oz vodka.
- 1 oz Wallingford Wanderlust strawberry-peppercorn marijuana syrup (approx. 20mg THC) *.
- 1 1/2 oz fresh-squeezed lemon juice.
- 1/2 oz straightforward syrup.
- 2-3 pieces cucumber.

Mushroom the cucumber in the shaker. Add the ice, vodka, syrup, primary as well as the lemon and drink until thoroughly chilled. Pour over the fresh ice in a highball glass, top with soda and garnish with the lemon and the cucumber pieces. Lemon slice and cucumber slice to garnish. NOTE: If you do not understand your tolerance, start with smaller sized quantities of marijuana syrup. Keep in mind that marijuana, as well as alcohol together, can affect you in a different way than either by itself. Never drive any vehicles under the influence of alcohol or marijuana.

Marijuana Milk (sugar-free).

Likewise called *Mother's Milk*, cannabis milk is the means several medical marijuana users decide to take their medicine. It is an excellent method to include marijuana right into your morning coffee or tea, as well as it's additionally an essential active ingredient in numerous marijuana beverages.

Right here is how to make it.

Active ingredients:

- Four mugs of whole milk.
- 1/4 ounce of finely ground marijuana flower.
- Cheesecloth.

Instructions:

Start by decarboxylating your marijuana in an oven readied to 240°. Spread the hash evenly on a baking sheet or recipe, and also cover with aluminium foil. Put it in the stove for twenty-five minutes, and also let it cool down. Utilising the double central heating boiler technique, bring the milk to a simmer. Add your marijuana gradually, mixing, up until the liquid covers the cannabis. Remove from heat, and also stress with a cheesecloth. Eject every decrease of milk from the cheesecloth to avoid squandering any one of the potent liquid. Permit to cool as well as delight in either alone or added to one more drink.

Vanilla Cannabis Milkshake.

It is among the new flexible cannabis beverage recipes that can be made use of to make any flavour of milkshake you desire switch to your recommended kind of gelato. Cannabis milk makes this a velvety, wonderful treat that is excellent for cooling you down on a hot day.

ingredients:

- 4 cups of vanilla ice cream.
- 1 3/4 cups of marijuana milk.
- 8 tablespoon sugar.
- 2 tsp vanilla extract.

Directions:

Incorporate active ingredients in a blender or food processor. Mix up until milkshake reaches preferred uniformity.

Pour into a high cooled glass and delight in.

Ingredients:

- 2/3 mugs sugar
- 3 1/4 cups water
- 1/2 mug lemon juice, newly pressed (about five lemons).
- 4-6 strawberries (tops cut off).
- 2 1/2 tablespoon fresh basil.
- Four tablespoon cannabis cast.

Directions:

Juice the lemons as well as set the juice aside in a big pitcher. Incorporate sugar with one mug of water in a small pan and bring to a boil. Stir frequently to ensure the sugar liquifies. Enable the combination to cool down at the space temperature level and also set in the refrigerator up until chilled. Add the syrup blend to the lemon juice, along with the marijuana cast, remaining water, strawberries, and also basil. Use an immersion mixer for regarding twenty secs to blend the active ingredients thoroughly. When the basil is delicately sliced, and the lemonade has transformed pink, it is prepared to be enjoyed. Offer chilled or over ice.

The only thing far better than enjoyable as well as creamy Thai iced tea? This tea that places the "high" in "Chai". Tip: keep a spoon or straw accessible to ensure the cannabutter remains correctly blended, and take pleasure in the benefits.

Ingredients:

- 6-8 Chai tea bags.
- Eight cups of boiling water.
- Mug of sugar.
- One can of sweetened condensed milk.
- 3-5 tbsps of melted cannabis butter.
-

Directions:

Steep tea bags in the steaming water for as regarding five minutes. Stir as well as eliminate pockets in the sugar. Incorporate condensed milk and cannabutter in a small bowl, and mix. Fill up glasses two-thirds of the means with tea and also include the butter mix to the top. It will sink, so make certain to have a straw or spoon helpful to blend it back in.

Active ingredients:

One of our favoured cannabis drinks, when the weather outside is terrible, this canna-cocoa dish is so beautiful. Work up a set of marijuana milk to make this chocolatey concoction, as well as you'll prepare to snuggle before the fire for hrs.

- 3/4 size mug of white sugar (alternative other sweeteners if wanted).
- One pinch of salt.
- a cup of boiling water.
- Three mugs of milk.
- 1/2 mugs of marijuana milk.
- 3/4 tsp of vanilla remove.
- 1/2 cup half-and-half.

Include salt, sugar, as well as cocoa to a saucepan. Gather the boiling water, and also offer a reduced boil while frequently stirring for concerning 2 mins.

Slowly include milk and marijuana milk while stirring. Warm until steaming, yet do not allow the liquid to reach a full boil or you'll run the risk of scalding. Eliminate from the heater, and also add vanilla. Split uniformly among a couple of mugs, and include half-and-half to cool.

When the cool of loss begins to work out in the air, nothing preferences far better than a mug of spiked hot apple cider. Except, that is, for this spiked warm apple cider that will get you high as the temperatures get reduced.

- 1 1/2 mugs Applejack or apple brandy.
- 1/4 cup of (pressed) light brown sugar. Three tablespoons of cannabutter.

- Six mugs of apple cider (or unfiltered apple juice).
- Six tablespoons fresh lemon juice.
- Six cinnamon sticks.
- Freshly grated nutmeg.

Directions:

In a large pot, bring cannabutter, brownish sugar, and applejack to a simmer over medium warmth. Mix frequently, as well as simmer up until the sugar, as well as butter, have both melted. Don't permit the combination to heat to the point of steaming, just simmering. Mix in cider, lemon juice, and also cinnamon sticks. Bring combination to a boil. Allow to steep for two or three minutes before offering. Garnish each cup with sprinkled nutmeg as well as a cinnamon stick.

Sparkling Pear Prosecco Canna Punch

ingredients:

Blend up a bowl of this pear prosecco strike if you're in the mood for a beverage that's as pretty as it is potent. Whether you're throwing a party, your chums won't neglect or searching for a pleasant porch-sipping drink for a silent night; this sparkling pink punch is an excellent, refreshing option amongst marijuana beverage dishes.

- Two components pear nectar or pear juice.
- Two components prosecco (for a non-alcoholic option, use gleaming cider or lemon-lime soda).
- 1 component cranberry juice.

- Ten mg-worth of marijuana tincture.
- Garnish with pear piece.

Cannabis-infused olive oil is a preferred among such distinguished Cannabis chefs as Doctor Diane. Depending upon the dose, this medication can severely disarm also one of the most skilled of Cannabis customers. The following is a to some extent adjusted version of Doctor Diane's renowned olive oil dish.

Components:

- 1/4 pounds dry bud or completely dry trimmings.
- Five mugs water (in the pot).
- Two mugs high-grade olive oil.
- Products:
- Pressure cooker or crockery pot.
- Grape press or extra-large coffee press pot.
- 1 Medium-length steel spoon.
- Latex handwear covers (not the ones with powder on them).
- Clean Container.
- Tidy Tupperware.
- High grape press filter or coffee filter.

Directions:

Place the five mugs of water in the pot and also offer a simmer (not a rolling boil). Add the two cups of oil as well as either 1/4 pound of completely dry bud or trimmings. Try not to stir, as the relocating water will certainly do this for you. Cover and turn the warm down to medium-low. You would prefer not to cook the water off since this aids in shielding your item from burning, and also hence to waste the THC. After 20 mins refuse the warmth altogether to low. After an additional 40 minutes (1 hr total amount) turn off the warm as well as remove the pressure cooker (or crockpot) from the heating surface. The remaining matter in the container ought to appear like wet mashed up grass cuttings with much of the liquid remaining. Next off, scoop the issue in your crockery pot or pressure cooker into your grape press or press pot. While you are doing this, guarantee that you spread out the matter evenly in journalism, so regarding getting optimal pushing ability. Put any continuing to be liquid into the press, as this is where the majority of the THC is focused. Heat two mugs of water and put it over what remains in the grape press or press pot. Make use of a fine filter and tighten this over your clean container with an elastic band or something comparable. Next off, begin the press the issue, slowly however progressively. The funnel from the grape press must be running into your clean container. The shade going through the pipe (if it is clear) must be dark green and also gold with some tan linked. Ensure you get all of the oil, as you won't want to waste one drop of this valuable medication (you might have to turn the press to get all of the liquid into your container. Squeeze out the filter over your box (this is where gloves are available in especially handy, as you can become extremely high from merely touching the mix) to obtain all of the oil. The oil needs to look like an inch or so deep layer on top with even more water below. Location this container in the freezer to strengthen overnight.

Incorporate pear and cranberry juices in a bottle or punch dish. Add cannabis cast, as well as delicately mix to blend.

Finish by pouring prosecco over the combination. Drift pear pieces on the top or usage as a garnish in each glass.

There is a cannabis-infused drink for every occasion if you know exactly how to make it. When you are taking in any mind-altering mixtures, remember to delight in responsibly continually.

- 3/4 mug THC olive oil
- Three grams kif (optional).
- One 15-ounce can garbanzo beans.
- 3/4 cup tahini (an essential active ingredient, discovered in the global area of the majority of grocery stores-- if not, try a Middle Eastern grocery store).
- 3 tbsps fresh lemon juice.
- 1/4 mug baked garlic, store-bought or homemade.
- Two tablespoons artichoke hearts drained well as well as chopped.
- 1/4 mug roasted red peppers, about sliced.
- 1 tsp freshly ground cumin seeds.
- One teaspoon salt.
- 1/2 tsp newly ground pepper.
- Pita bread, warmed up in the oven, for the offering.
- In a little saucepan, cosy your THC olive oil over a reduced heat. Remove from warm.
- 2. Place the garbanzo beans, tahini, lemon juice, roasted garlic, artichoke hearts, red peppers, cumin, and 1/2 cup of the cosy THC oil in a portion of food.
- Gradually include more oil as needed. Include the salt and also pepper.

ENVIRONMENT-FRIENDLY LEAFY KALE SALAD IN BROWN CANNABUTTER

VINAIGRETTE

Dish

Kale is among the most healthy things you can consume, so make sure to include even more of it in your diet regimen, especially when doused with this decadent clothing from our buddy chef Bobby Hellen. Chef Hellen uses this vinaigrette on a comparable salad at the dining establishment, absent the individual component. It makes clothing for more than one salad as well as maintains for an extended period in the fridge.

- ROCKS 2.
- SALAD.
- One extra pound Tuscan kale.
- 1/2 cup slivered almonds.
- VINAIGRETTE.
- 1/3 cup saltless butter.
- 1/3 mug Simple Cannabutter (see recipe).
- 1/3 mug sherry vinegar or red wine vinegar can be replaced.
- Salt.

1. Clean kale, remove centre stalks, and also roughly cut the leaves into bite-size pieces.

2. Toast almonds in a dry sauté pan over medium warmth, drinking the frying pot periodically up until you smell the almonds, concerning 5 mins. Remove from warmth.

3. To make the vinaigrette, in a small saucepan, thaw the saltless butter over high heat until browned, then include the cannabutter, only up until melted.

Get rid of warm. Add the sherry vinegar and also period with a pinch or more of salt.

4. Outfit the kale with 4 to 6 tbsps of clothing, throw with the almonds, as well as offer cosy.

When you draw the container out of your freezer the following day, you ought to have a tidy Tupperware (or similar container) close by. Use a metal spoon to remove the strengthened yet slightly doughy (it resembles Play-Doh) combination as well as area it in your box. The mix should be a light, environment-friendly shade. Any brown issue you see is water, and as much of this as feasible must be removed. Once you have successfully accumulated every one of this valuable mix, it will be ready to medicate with. Shop it in the fridge freezer, or it will go wrong. Warning: 1/2 mug of this olive oil is equivalent to 1 ounce of marijuana. Use properly for your details needs. This good reward is celebrated to spread out on toasted bread, use in several of your favoured food preparation recipes, as well as even makes for an exceptionally effective topical medication.

STUFFED STONED JALAPEÑO POPPERS

When a particularly durable jalapeño pepper plant expanded on my New York City rooftop ruptured forth with a bounty of twenty peppers, these stoner deals with were born. While partaking of a great joint as well as relaxing on the same rooftop, inspiration struck: peppers, peanut butter, as well as a pot! The peanut butter tempers the warmth of the peppers, and the natural herb obtains you high-- what extra can you request for from something this straightforward to make? To amuse your bouche as well as attempt these one-bite wonders

- Ten jalapeño peppers
- Two tablespoons THC Oil (see recipe).
- 1/4 cup eco-friendly onions, white parts only, sliced.
- Two cloves garlic, minced.
- 3/4 cup peanut butter.

1. Use a small blade to get rid of as much of the pith and seeds as possible Peppers that can hold the padding.

2. Rinsing out within the pepper with water is a great way to eliminate the seeds.

3. Warm a little saucepan over tool warmth and also include the THC Oil. Allow the oil cosy for concerning 30 seconds, after that include the green onions and even cook for 1 minute.

4. Then add the garlic and also sauté for 1 to 2 minutes. Add the peanut butter and also stir, adding 2 to 3 tablespoons water as required to thin the.

Uniformity. The sauce needs to be simple to mix. Eliminate from warmth.

Use a spoon, piping bag, or a tiny funnel to fill the jalapeños with the peanut butter sauce. Fit the pepper covers back on and also protect with a. Toothpick.

5. Area peppers on a foil-lined cooking sheet and even cook for 20 minutes. Serve cosy.

Note: You may want handwear covers to take care of the peppers, yet if you don't put on gloves, beware not to touch your eyes after taking care of the peppers. Laundry your hands as well as the reducing board right away and extensively after handling peppers.

A dish from Chef Bliss.

Cook Bliss developed these springtime rolls for a tasting menu that was offered to the High Times staff in New York. Each dish on that amazing buffet was sautéed in, brushed with, or otherwise instilled with cannabis butter and oil. These sativa shrimp spring rolls would undoubtedly benefit from using a strain such as Haze, with a terpene account that will undoubtedly match the Asian flavours.

- MANGO SAUCE.
- One mango, peeled off and also diced.
- One clove garlic, finely sliced.
- One tablespoon sugar.
- 1 tbsp coarsely chopped ginger.
- 1/2 little habanero pepper, seeded and carefully chopped.
- 1/4 mug orange juice.
- Two tablespoons of rice white wine vinegar.
- One teaspoon THC Oil (see dish).
- SPRING ROLLS.
- 1/2 mug plus 3 tbsps THC Oil (see dish).
- 1/4 cup cut shiitake mushrooms.

- One teaspoon plus two tablespoons soy sauce.
- One teaspoon sesame oil.
- One tablespoon sliced garlic.
- 1 tbsp cut shallot.
- 1/3 cup julienned or shredded carrots.
- 1/3 cup julienned red and also yellow bell peppers (an even mix of both shades).
- 1/2 napa cabbage, shredded.
- Two tablespoons Asian chilli paste.
- 2 tsp lime juice.
- 2 tbsps cut environment-friendly onions.
- 1 tbsp cut ginger.
- 2 tbsp chopped cilantro.
- 2 tsp salt, plus more to taste.
- Two teaspoons black pepper, plus more to taste.
- One pound rock shrimp, cleaned and also deveined.
- One 12-ounce plan spring roll wrappers.
- One egg.
- 1/2 cup cornstarch.

1. To make the mango sauce, in a tool pan over high warmth, integrate mango, garlic, sugar, ginger, habanero, orange juice, and rice wine vinegar. Bring to a boil, then simmer over reduced heat for 5 minutes. Get rid of warmth and allow it to cool.

2. In a blender or food processor, combine the mango mix with THC Oil and also blend till smooth. Set aside.

3. To make the spring rolls, in a small fry pan, heat 1 tbsp of the THC Oil above. Add mushrooms and also cook till golden brownish, then add one teaspoon of the soy sauce as well as one teaspoon of the sesame oil. Transfer to a dish and also set aside.

4. Reheat the frying pan over high warmth and include one tablespoon of the THC Oil. When the oil is hot, add the garlic, shallot, carrots, bell peppers, as well as a cabbage as well as sauté for 1 minute, then include the chilli paste, two tablespoons of the soy sauce, the lime juice, green onions, ginger, and cilantro. Drain veggies in a filter (if you leave the liquid in when the springtime roll is fried, it will blow up) and also season with salt and even black pepper. Allot.

5. Reheat the pan over high heat and also add 1 tbsp of the THC oil. Eliminate from warmth, drainpipe, slice approximately, as well as a season with a pinch of salt as well as pepper.

6. To set up, outlined your springtime roll wrapper diagonally, with an edge directing towards you, so it appears like a diamond form. Blend the egg, as well as comb a thin layer onto the spring roll wrapper.

7. Spread 2 tbsps of the dental filling in the middle of the wrapper and also bring the bottom corner of the wrapper over the mixture, after that fold in the sides and also roll upward, making the roll as tight as you can. Roll in the cornstarch on a plate as well as allowed. Repeat with continuing to be filling as well as wrappers.

Do not crowd the frying pan; fry only a few rolls at a time so you can transform them quickly. Drain on paper towels and also serve with the mango sauce.

Guacamole is a healthy and balanced reward that every person enjoys, and also when you include a dash of THC

Oil, you'll obtain the party started! Offer this dip with Mini Kind Veggie Burritos, or devour with a bag of chips.

- Four ripe avocados, peeled off and pits eliminated, one pit booked
- One cucumber, peeled with seeds removed, diced
- 1/2 cup sliced eco-friendly onions, environment-friendly and white parts
- Two cloves garlic, diced
- 1/2 mug THC Oil (see dish).
- One jalapeno pepper.
- 1/2 cup securely loaded cilantro, cut.
- Juice of 2 limes.
- One teaspoon salt.

Combine all the active ingredients in a food processor as well as mix until the texture is smooth. Keep the reserved avocado pit in the offering bowl with the guac, as it will certainly aid keep it fresh and also protect against browning. Refrigerate any remaining guacamole in an airtight container with cling wrap covering the surface area. Use within one day.

MINI KIND VEGGIE BURRITOS

The Kind Veggie Burrito has its origins in Mexican food; however, it became a locoweed tale in America using the Grateful Dead vehicle parking whole lot scene. Easy to prepare in advance of time, inexpensive to make, and also sold at a high-enough markup to high-enough jam-band followers, these burritos might fund a cross-country adventure. Enhance the appetiser by dipping the little burritos right into ganja-oil guacamole, offer two or three as an entrée, or make normal-size burritos.

- One 15-ounce can vegetarian refried beans.
- One 15-ounce can black beans, drained pipes and also washed.
- 6 tbsps THC Oil, plus a lot more for brushing (see recipe).
- One sweet onion, diced.
- One little zucchini or summer season squash, shredded.
- 2 tsp salt.
- One red bell pepper, chopped.
- One mug sliced mushrooms.
- One cup diced fit to be tied potatoes (or leftover roasted potatoes).
- One teaspoon paprika.
- Two teaspoons cumin.
- 1/4 teaspoon cayenne pepper.
- One mug prepared long-grain brown rice.
- Twenty little flour tortillas (soft taco dimension).
- Two cups shredded cheddar cheese.
- Salsa, sour lotion, and Ganja Guacamole (see recipe), for the offering.

1. Preheat the oven to 300 ° F. 2. In a 2-quart pot, mix the two containers of beans along with 2 to 3 tbsps of water, and give a simmer over low heat.

2. While the beans are cooking, warm a sauté frying pan over medium heat and also include six tablespoons THC Oil. Allow the oil cosy for thirty seconds, then add the onion and also sauté till golden brown, concerning eight minutes.

3. While the onion is cooking, throw the shredded zucchini with 1 tsp salt in a colander as well as squeeze out the excess water. Allot.

4. Include the bell pepper to the sautéed onions and cook for a couple of mins before adding the zucchini, mushrooms, as well as potatoes. Get rid of vegetable mix from the warmth and include the staying 1 tsp salt.

5. Place one heaping dose of veggies as well as rice in the middle, topped by a little spray of cheese. To fold up, bring the lower edge of the tortilla up over the filling, then put the sides in and cover with the leading edge of the tortilla.

6. You desire a self-contained package with as little filling up befalling as feasible. The area of the burrito in a glass baking frying pan, as well as repeat up until you have twenty little burritos or until you, run out of filling up.

7. Brush the burritos with THC Oil, and bake for ten minutes, just up until the tortillas are golden brown. Serve with salsa, sour cream, as well as Ganja Guacamole.

Dish submitted by a man from Texas.

Very first sent by a visitor from South Texas. These nachos couldn't be simpler to make, can't potentially be screwed up, but can likely fuck you up if you consume way too much. Serve these up in your male cave the following time you invite your bromantic buddies over for Texas Hold 'em, the Super Bowl, or only an incredible dish.

- Two red tomatoes.
- One eco-friendly plant.
- One large pleasant onion.

- One jalapeño or serrano pepper.
- Two cloves garlic, minced.
- Three tablespoons beer (a light beer like Bud or Corona).
- 3 tbsps fresh lemon juice.
- 3 tbsps THC Oil (see recipe).
- 6 ounces tortilla chips.
- One cup shredded Monterey Jack cheese.
- One ripe avocado, diced.

1. Preheat the oven to 350 ° F.

2. Roughly slice the tomatoes, onion, as well as jalapeño, and add to a food processor. Add the garlic, beer, lemon juice, and THC Oil. Pulse 2 or 3 times to incorporate, maintaining the texture beefy.

3. Spread out the chips on a baking sheet, cover with the cheese, as well as top with numerous heaping spoonfuls of the pico de hashish you made.

PESTO

- Three tablespoons walnuts, sliced.
- Two cups basil, firmly packed.
- Pinch sea salt.
- Two cloves garlic, minced.
- 1/4 cup fresh grated Parmesan cheese.
- 1/2 to 3/4 mug THC olive oil (see dish).

BRUSCHETTA

- One big loaf ciabatta bread, cut into 1-inch-thick slices.
- 3 tbsps THC olive oil (see recipe).

- 2 or 3 antique or natural farmers' market tomato, sliced.
- Medicated Balsamic Vinegar (optional).

A staple in Italian food preparation, basil radiates in pesto, a sauce coming from in the Genoa region, not together residence to a world-famous pressure of basil. When storing, regularly cover the surface area with a thin layer of oil and also plastic wrap to maintain it from turning brownish. If you would like to try pairing specific cannabis stress with basil, use Genovese basil and also look for ganja with a citrusy fragrance, indicating the existence of limonene, a terpene likewise located in basil plants.

Marijuana Pancakes

- Active ingredients:
- Two mugs all-round flour
- 2 1/2 tsp cooking powder
- 1/2 tsp salt
- One egg, beaten gently
- 1 1/2 cups milk
- 2 tbsp weed butter, thawed

Instructions:

1. Filter together the first three components (to prevent lumps).

2. In a separate bowl, mix egg and also milk, then add it to the flour mix, stirring up until merely smooth.

3. Mix in weed butter.

* Note: If you intend to mix it up, throw in blueberries, a little dice of apple, or small bits of banana.

4. Grease a skillet or nonstick pot with cooking spray or a little grease.

5. Heat pan on medium for concerning ten minutes.

6. Pour batter to make pancakes of whatever size you such as.

7. Cook first side up until bubbles base on top, concerning 3 minutes; then turn as well as prepare another hand till it, also, is brownish, about two minutes.

8. Serve quickly with weed butter and syrup or hold briefly in the cosy oven.

9. Inform us regarding your experience in a remark below once you have learned exactly how to make marijuana pancakes and also have consumed them!

MEAT LOAF

Ingredients:

- 2 lbs. Ground beef (or ground meat of your choice).

- 1/2 oz. Carefully ground marijuana.
- One nicely chopped onion.
- One sliced tomato.
- One chopped stick celery.
- One egg.
- Four pieces salute (fallen apart into bread crumbs).

Instructions:

Mix all the components in a large dish. Make sure the meat you utilise has a respectable amount of fat in it, as you will certainly require it for the THC to be appropriately triggered by the warm as well as taken in by the fat and also egg.

Cannabis Spinach

Ingredients:

- 1/3 cup cannabis-infused olive oil.
- One lot of spinach.Five cloves garlic, minced.
- 1 tsp sriracha sauce (or chilli powder).
- 2 tbsp oyster sauce.
- 1 tsp black pepper.
- Salt to taste.

Directions:

Warmth the cannabis-infused olive oil in a large saucepan on reduced. Include the garlic and cook for two mins, mixing. Include in the chilli sauce, oyster sauce, salt as well as pepper and stir till mixed.

Ingredients:

- One defrosted salmon fillet, 1 pound.
- 8 grams of cannabis.
- Two cloves garlic, diced.
- One huge onion, cut.
- 1 tsp pepper.
- One tomato, very finely sliced.
- Three tablespoon dry bread crumbs.
- 1 tbsp vegetable oil (Optional: replace with marijuana olive oil).

Directions:

Grind up the marijuana with a coffee mill till it becomes a fine powder. Mix with dry bread crumbs as well as set aside. Spray a shallow cooking frying pan with non-stick covering. Place the fish in the baking pan and also spray with pepper, garlic as well as oregano. Layer with tomato pieces as well as onion. Mix bread crumbs with oil as well as placed a layer on top of the fish. Bake at 350° for around twelve-fifteen minutes or only until fish flakes quickly. Four portions.

Ingredients:

- 2/3 cup cannabis-infused olive oil.
- 1 1/3 mug catsup.
- 1/2 cup water.
- 1/4 mug white sugar.
- One tablespoon brown sugar.

- 1 tbsp merlot vinegar.
- 1 tbsp prepared yellow mustard.
- 1 tsp salt.
- 1/4 tsp ground black pepper.
- 1/4 tsp paprika.
- 2 pounds hamburger.
- 2 tsp minced onion.
- Two tablespoon soy sauce.
- Burger buns.

Directions:

Mix the ketchup, water, cannabis-infused olive oil, white sugar, brown sugar, vinegar, mustard, salt, pepper, as well as paprika in a large pan over low warmth. In a different big pot, cook and mix the ground soy, onion as well as beef sauce over medium-high warm up until the beef is browned as well as fully cooked. Mix the meat into the cosy sauce, as well as heat with each other on reduced for ten minutes.

Cannabis Balsamic Vinaigrette

Components:

- 3/4 cup extra-virgin marijuana olive oil
- 3/4 cup balsamic vinegar
- Two finely minced cloves of garlic
- 2 tsp. dijon-style mustard (optional).
- 1/2 tsp. oregano.
- Pinch of salt.
- Pinch of pepper.

Instructions:

Now for the challenging component: place all the active ingredients in a blender or food processor as well as mix until extensively combined. Store in mason jars in the fridge.

Ingredients:

- 3 or 4 pieces of yellow squash.
- 1/3 mug cannabis-infused olive oil.
- Six cloves garlic, diced.
- Two tablespoon soy sauce.
- One tablespoon garlic powder.
- 1 tsp chilli powder.
- Salt and pepper to taste.

Instructions:

Warmth the marijuana olive oil in a big pan on really reduced. Cut the squash into 1/4 inch slices and also dice the garlic. Place the squash, garlic, soy sauce, garlic powder, chilli powder, salt and pepper right into the cannabis olive oil. Do not permit oil to steam. Sautee on low till the squash becomes soft, overcooking permits it to soak up more oil. Transfer the squash to a dish as well as drain pipes the remaining oil right into a container to conserve in the fridge for the next batch. Makes three portions.

Ingredients:

- 1/3 cup cannabis-infused olive oil.

- One plan spaghetti.
- One whole light bulb garlic, chopped.
- Two tablespoon vegetable oil.
- 1 tbsp soy sauce.
- Parmesan cheese.
- Salt and pepper to preference.

Directions:

In an enormous pot bring water to a bubble. Cook the pasta to desired tenderness. In the interim, dice the garlic as well as sautee it in the grease and soy sauce over medium warmth until delicate. Transform the heat to reduced and also include cannabis olive oil. Temperature for five minutes and after that reserved. Toss the noodles right into the oil and mix in pepper, parmesan as well as salt cheese to preference.

Marijuana Pepper and Artichoke Dip

Ingredients:

- Two tablespoons mighty marijuana butter.
- Two jars seasoned artichoke hearts (6.5 oz).
- One leek, diced.
- Three tablespoon mayo.
- One jar roasted red peppers (7 oz).
- 3/4 cup grated parmesan cheese.

Instructions:

In a medium saucepan, soften the cannabis spread slowly on low warmth. Stir in the artichoke hearts, heated red peppers, parmesan cheese and mayonnaise. Offer with warmed up Cannabis Flat Bread or tortilla chips.

Ingredients:

- 8 oz. medicated olive oil.
- 30 oz. Water.
- Two peeled off and also diced tomatoes.
- Eight chopped pieces of bacon.
- Three big peeled as well as sliced potatoes.
- Four sliced garlic cloves.
- One big cut yellow onion.
- Ten peppercorns.
- Three bay leaves.
- Salt to taste.

Instructions:

Heat all ingredients (except potatoes) in a massive pot for fifteen minutes. After the total amount of fourty-five minutes is up, add the sliced and also peeled off potatoes and continue cooking for another fourty-five minutes.

Cannabis Alfredo Pasta Sauce

Ingredients:

- 1/2 stick (1/4 cup) cannabutter.
- One cup of heavy cream (usage medicated milk recipe on cream for an even more powerful sauce).
- Two cloves garlic (minced).
- Oregano to taste.
- 1.5 cup fresh-grated Parmesan or Gruyere cheese.
- 1/4 mug fresh chopped parsley.

Instructions:

First, thaw the cannabutter in a saucepan on medium to low warmth. Include the heavy cream (ideally medicated) and also simmer at the same temperature for five minutes. Include the cheese, garlic as well as oregano as well as stir or blend quickly, while leaving the heat on a tool to low. One minute before you are ready to serve, mix in the parsley as well as pour over your favoured pasta of a medicated as well as savoury treat.

Marijuana Chili

Ingredients:

- 1 oz. Finely ground marijuana buds (usage low-grade or mid buds if you do not desire it to be also expensive).
- 2 pounds. Ground beef.
- 46 oz. Tomato juice.
- 40 oz. Tomato sauce.
- Two cups onion (sliced).
- 1/2 cup green bell pepper (sliced).
- 1/2 mug celery (cut).
- 1/2 cup mushrooms (sliced).
- 1/4 mug chilli powder.
- Two mugs beans of your option.
- 2 tsp. Cumin.
- 1 tsp. Salt.
- Three cloves of garlic (diced).
- 1/2 tsp. black pepper (ground).
- 1/2 tsp. oregano.
- 1/2 tsp. sugar.
- 1/2 tsp. chilli pepper.

Directions:

Place two pounds of beef in frying pan or skillet and brownish over medium or medium-high heat. Once it is completely browned, drainpipe extensively as well as set aside. Put all ingredients except for ground cannabis in a considerable pot and also offer a steady boil. After it pertains to a boil, decrease warm to low-medium and also place in the ground cannabis. Cook for one to two hours, minimising the warmth to low after one hour. Serve and even enjoy.

Ingredients.

- 4 tbsp. (half-stick) Cannabutter.
- 5.25 mugs rye bread crumbs (or any unseasoned bread crumbs).
- 1/2 mug cut celery.
- 1 cup almonds/cashews (finely chopped).
- 1/3 cup carefully cut onions.
- Two tablespoons. Chicken seasoning (steak spices for duck).
- Two tablespoons. Red wine.
- 1/2 Wheatgrass / chives cup sliced.

Directions:

Melt butter over low heat on a stovetop or in the microwave at low temperature (this is to make sure that you do not compromise the effectiveness. THC can survive temperatures as much as 385 levels Fahrenheit).

Once the cannabutter has been thawed, mix all the components and stuff in the bird before cooking.

Ingredients:

- As numerous romaine lettuce leaves as you desire
- 4 prepared as well as squashed strips of bacon
- Croutons
- Three tablespoons. grated parmesan cheese
- 2 tbsp. cannabis olive oil
- 2 tbsp. mayo
- One clove garlic (diced).
- 2 tsp. White vinegar.
- 1 tsp. Dijon mustard.
- 1 tsp. Anchovy paste (optional, but essential for a TRUE caesar salad).
- 1/4 tsp. Worcestershire sauce.
- 1/4 tsp. salt.
- 1/4 tsp. ground black pepper.

Directions:

For the clothing, mix the cannabis olive oil, 2 tsp. For the salad, cut the romaine lettuce right into bite-size items and place it in a tool or large salad dish. Currently include the croutons, bacon as well as the last tablespoon.

Instructions:

Okay, this one is straightforward, yet equally as potent as cannabutter or olive oil, if used in baked goods or any recipe asking for flour. Pick off all the stems as well as seeds (with any luck there are not any type of) as well as put the buds into a coffee mill, grinding until the buds become a fine powder, similar in uniformity to that of regular flour. Remain to do this up until you have as much flour as you require. Substitute this canna flour for versatile flour in any dish. Bear in mind to keep the temperature at 380 degrees Fahrenheit or reduced, so you do not destroy the cannabinoids.

Components:

- Two tablespoon cannabis butter.
- 3 tbsp cannabis butter, thawed.
- Twenty-four entire fresh mushrooms, small to tool dimension.
- One environment-friendly onion, minced.
- 1 tsp lemon juice.
- One mug cooked crab meat, diced.
- 1/2 cup soft bread crumbs.
- One egg, beaten with a fork.
- 1/2 tsp dry dill weed.
- 3/4 mug shredded pepper jack cheese.
- 1/4 mug completely dry white wine.
- a couple of leaves basil, cut into thin strips.

Instructions:

Warmth stove to 350. Put the 3 tbsp thawed butter into a 13 X 9 steel frying pan. Eliminate the stems from the mushrooms as well as set the caps apart. Carefully chop up the remaining stems. Thaw the 2 tbsp butter in a medium saucepan and also cook the onion and mushroom together for concerning 3 minutes. Eliminate from warm as well as mix in the lemon juice, crab, soft bread crumbs, egg, dill weed and 1/4 cup of the pepper jack cheese. The area the mushroom caps right into the baking frying pan, as well as mix them around up until covered in the cannabis butter. Arrange the caps with the cavity side up, and also stuff kindly with the crab mix. Complete with the remaining 1/2 mug of cheese, and pour them a glass of wine into the pan around the mushrooms (out the top). Bake for fifteen-twenty-five mins, until the cheese, is melted as well as a little browned. I am leading with the sliced basil and also delight in!

Marijuana Flour.

Ingredients:

As numerous marijuana buds (absolutely no stems or seeds) as you desire to make flour out of.

Cannabis Olivia

Active ingredients:

- 1/3 cup cannabis olive oil.
- 3/4 pounds. Matched olives.
- Two cloves fresh minced garlic.
- Pepper to taste.

Directions:

Place the garlic, olives and marijuana olive oil in a blender or food processor, blending up until smooth. If it comes out runny, include even more olives. Put the pasta in a pot or container and also mix in pepper. Put in a mason container, pour a slim layer of marijuana olive oil on the leading as well as store in the refrigerator. Spread on your favoured sourdough bread, include in egg meals and even baked potatoes.

Ingredients:

- One pound pasta, preferably spiral or bowtie.
- Four Roma tomatoes.
- Five cloves garlic, diced.
- 3/4 mug cannabis-infused olive oil.
- Fresh basil.
- Salt and pepper to taste.

Directions:

Mince the garlic, as well as cut the basil into strips. Include the cannabis-infused olive pepper, oil and salt and mix in. Makes four substantial servings.

Components:

- Two sticks salty cannabutter
- 1/4 mug cream cheese
- 1 cup flour
- One tool egg
- Pepper as well as dill to taste
- One cup experienced bread crumbs (Italian flavouring seems to work finest).
- Peanut oil to deep fry balls in.

Directions:

Thoroughly mix cannabutter, cream pepper, cheese and dill in an electric mixer. Next off, making use of either a tiny spoon or melon spoon, form the mixture into different 1-inch spheres as well as a place on an item of wax paper on a baking sheet. Take pleasure in, but be cautious, only one or two of these will medicate you, even if your butter is of average potency.

Active ingredients:

- One extra pound poultry breast, boneless and skinless and diced right into dices.
- 1 3/4 mug poultry broth/stock.
- 1 cup eco-friendly peas.
- One mug diced carrots.
- 1/2 mug diced celery.
- 2/3 cup 2% milk.
- 1/3 cup cannabutter.
- 1/3 mug diced onion.
- 1/3 mug flour.
- 1/2 tsp. salt.
- 1/4 tsp. crushed black pepper.
- 1/4 tsp. Celery seed.
- Two 9-inch unbaked pie crusts.

Instructions:

In a frying pan, integrate the poultry items, peas, carrots and also celery and add 1/3 mug water, cover and boil for fifteen minutes over medium-high warmth. Presently, in the same skillet, cook the onions in margarine (either cannabutter or ordinary spread) till they are soft and start the come to be precise. Utilize a spread cutting edge to diminish about six slits in the leading to empower wetness and substantial steam to escape. To make this distinctive edible, include your very own Cannabis-infused butter to any homemade macaroni as well as cheese recipe or even a boxed macaroni and cheese container. Whenever it calls for butter, obviously substitute the medicated butter for regular. When you have the butter made, the entire procedure takes much less than fifteen minutes, making it one of the fastest means to make a medicated dish. Additionally, as a result of the reality that the recipe typically does not require too much butter, it is an excellent idea to make your Cannabis-infused butter more potent than you generally would. It merely relies on your individual preference.

Potatoe Mash.

Ingredients:

- 1/2 to 1 stick cannabis butter, depending upon effectiveness.
- Four large potatoes, peeled.
- One bunch of garlic.
- One cup shredded cheddar cheese.
- 1/2 mug sour cream.
- Salt, pepper to preference.
- A dashboard of olive oil (to roast garlic).

Directions:

You will certainly want to prepare the roasted garlic. Cut the top off of the lot as well as for drizzle regarding a tablespoon of olive oil right into the garlic. Include the cannabis butter, allowing to blend and thaw in wholly. Add the sour cream, cheese, baked garlic, salt and pepper and mix with each other. For a delicious as well as special marijuana recipe, spread this pesto on your favourite bread, crackers or as a substitute for pesto pasta.

Active ingredients:

- 1/3 mug medicated extra-virgin olive oil.
- One cup chopped fresh cilantro with or without stems.
- 1/2 mug sun-dried tomatoes.
- One clove of minced fresh garlic.
- One tablespoon. Carefully cut eco-friendly chiles or fresh jalapeño.
- 1 tsp. Brown sugar.
- Salt and pepper as favoured.

Directions:

It's not essential, yet if time authorisations, soak the sun-dried tomatoes in the olive oil for at least two hours. After they have soaked, blend the cilantro, tomatoes, chile or jalapeño, olive oil, garlic, and darker sugar till entirely blended. Get, delight in as well as serve. You can store it in the ice chest for as long as two days.

CANNABIS PIZZA

The reason why is clear: not only is it an excellent method to medicate, the majority of pizzas are adequate to qualify as a dish for individuals. A much a lot more rewarding experience can be making your own medicated pizza.

Makes two pizzas.

Ingredients:

- Dough:
- 3 1/2 mugs flour.
- 1 oz. Yeast.
- 1 tsp yeast.
- Eight fl. oz. Water.
- One tablespoon granulated sugar.
- Two tablespoons thawed CannaButter (potency depends upon the dose of your butter).
- Toppings:
- Two cups grated cheese of your selection.
- One large can of sliced tomatoes.
- 2 tsp freshly ground oregano.
- Any other desired toppings.
- Five tablespoons thawed CannaButter.

Guidelines:

Include the flour, yeast as well as sugar in a large mixing dish. Add water and continuously blend it right into the dough. Uncover, adding the salt as well as two tablespoons of melted CannaButter, and also mix right into a mixture round. You are ultimately adding the cheese as well as any more toppings you want. Cook in the oven for thirteen to eighteen minutes.

Cannabis Salsa N Papaya

Active ingredients

- Two mugs diced papaya
- 1/2 red onion, diced
- One red bell pepper, diced
- 1/4 cup sliced fresh cilantro
- 2 tbsps lime juice
- One clove garlic, minced

- 1/4 tsp hot chile paste, or to taste
- 4 (6 ounces) tuna steaks
- 1/4 mug THC oil
- salt and pepper to taste
- Three eggs
- 1/2 cup cut macadamia nuts

Directions

Integrate the papaya, onion, and also red pepper in a dish. Include the cilantro, lime juice, garlic, and warm chile paste. Throw to combine, then cool until prepared to serve. Preheat a grill flame broil for high warm, as well as lightly oil grind. Brush the fish steaks with olive oil, at that point period with salt and pepper. Dunk the fish steaks in the egg, and furthermore license excess egg to run off. Prepare the tuna steaks on the preheated grill to your desired level of doneness, concerning two minutes per side for medium. Offer with the papaya salsa.

Cannabis Salmon

Active ingredients

- 1 1/2 extra pounds salmon fillets
- lemon pepper to preference
- garlic powder to liking
- salt to taste
- 1/3 cup soy sauce
- 1/3 mug brownish sugar
- 1/3 cup water
- 1/4 mug THC oil

Instructions

Season salmon filets with lemon pepper, garlic powder, and salt.

In a little dish, stir with one another soy sauce, dark colored sugar, water, and furthermore vegetable oil until sugar is liquified. Spot fish in a substantial resealable plastic sack with the soy sauce combination, seals, and even resort to cover. Refrigerate for in any event two hours. Preheat grill for tool warmth. Lightly oil grill grate. Location salmon on the preheated grill, and discard marinade. Prepare salmon for six to eight minutes per side, or till the fish flakes quickly with a fork.

Marijuana Salmon Mapple

Active ingredients

- 1/4 cup maple syrup
- Two tablespoons soy sauce
- One clove garlic, minced
- 1/4 teaspoon garlic salt
- 1/8 teaspoon ground black pepper
- 1 pound salmon
- Two tablespoons weed butter

Instructions

In a little bowl, blend the maple syrup, soy sauce, garlic, garlic salt, and pepper. Area salmon in a shallow glass cooking dish, and layer with the maple syrup blend. Cover the recipe, as well as season salmon in the fridge thiry minutes, transforming when. Preheat stove to 400 levels F (200 levels C).

Place the cooking recipe in the preheated oven, and also bake salmon exposed twenty minutes, or up until easily flaked with a fork. Melt weed butter on salmon when completed cooking.

Active ingredients

- Two extra pounds tilapia fillets
- 2 tbsps lime juice
- 2 tsp salt
- 1 tsp ground black pepper
- 1 tsp garlic powder
- One teaspoon paprika
- cooking spray
- Two tablespoons of weed butter
- 1/2 cup plain fat-free yoghurt
- 2 tbsps lime juice
- 1 1/2 tablespoons chopped fresh cilantro
- 1 1/2 teaspoons tinned chipotle peppers in adobo sauce
- 16 (5 inches) corn tortillas
- Two mugs shredded cabbage
- 1 cup shredded Monterey Jack cheese
- One tomato, cut
- One avocado - peeled off, matched, and cut
- 1/2 cup salsa
- Two environment-friendly onions, chopped

Directions

Rub tilapia fillets with two tablespoons lime juice as well as a season with salt, black pepper, garlic powder, and also paprika. Spray both sides of each net with cooking spray. Preheat grill for medium

Baked Cannabis Tilapia

Active ingredients

- 4 (4 ounce) fillets tilapia
- Two teaspoons weed butter
- 1/4 tsp Old Bay Seasoning TM, or to taste
- 1/2 tsp garlic salt, or to taste
- One lemon, sliced up
- 1 (16 ounces) package frozen cauliflower with broccoli and also red pepper

Instructions

Preheat the stove to 375 degrees F (190 degrees F). Oil a 9x13 inch baking dish. Period with Old Bay flavouring and also garlic salt. Set up the frozen mixed vegetables around the fish, as well as period lightly with salt and even pepper. Cover the meal and bake for twenty-five to thirty minutes in the preheated oven, until vegetables hurt and also fish flakes conveniently with a fork.

Cannabis Hash Brown Casserole

Active ingredients:

* concerning 1/2 bundle of icy hash browns

* 4 or 5 eggs

* concerning 1/4 pound of your preferred cheese: shredded, grated, or tremendously finely cut

* (Optional) Grits and also salsa and Tobasco, and so on

* 2 Tablespoons of weed butter

Directions:

Add the 2 tbsps of weed butter into a big skillet. Include hash browns, mixing so the oil layers most of them. Brown the potatoes for about six or eight minutes, occasionally mixing, until an all-time low of the pile starts looking gold. As vegetables are browning, defeat the eggs as well as a slice or grate celebrity, if essential. When the potatoes are lightly golden on the bottom, turn the potato patty over as cleanly as possible, and also put the eggs over the top. Permit this side to brown until the eggs are mostly strengthened, around five or eight minutes. Now flip the mixture over again, as quickly as possible, and after that, prepare the cheese in a thin layer on top. Cover the frying pan preferably and also permit the cheese to thaw (around eight or ten minutes, much less if covered). Offer with salsa and grits.

Marijuana Baked Pizza Sandwich

ingredients:

- 1 lb Lean Ground Beef
- 15 oz Tomatos Sauce; 1 Cn, OR 15 oz Pizza Sauce 1 Cn
- One ts Oregano Leaves

- 2 c Biscuit Baking Mix
- One ea Egg; Lg
- 2/3 c weed Milk
- 8 oz Cheese; *

- 2 oz Mushrooms; Sliced, Drained,1 Cn.
- 1/4 c Parmesan Cheese; Grated.

Prep work:

* Use one 8-oz package of chopped procedure American Or mozzarella cheese. Method out 3/4 cup of the batter as well as set aside. Layer 4 pieces of the cheese, the meat mixture, the mushrooms as well as the continuing to be cheese on top of the batter and also tomato sauce.

Marijuana BBQ Beef Sandwiches

Ingredients:

- 3 pounds beef chuck
- Two onions, sliced
- 1 (28 ounces) can cut up tomatoes, with juice
- 1/2 cup distilled white vinegar
- 1/2 mug water
- Three tablespoons sugar
- 1/3 (10 liquid ounce) bottle Worcestershire sauce
- salt and pepper to preference
- 2 tbsps of weed butter

Preparation:

Place roast in a Dutch stove, and also spray with chopped onions. Cover with tomatoes, water, sugar as well as Worcestershire sauce. Period with salt and pepper. Cook over tool warm with lid a little ajar for three hours. Remove meat, as well as shred with two forks. Dispose of bones, fat as well as cartilage. Place shredded beef back into the sauce, and cook till liquid is lowered, fifteen to twenty minutes. Apply weed butter as wanted

INDGREDIENTS:

- 1 pound campanile or Gemelli noodles
- 1 pound (regarding two large) boneless, skinless chicken busts, cubed
- 1/2 mug breadcrumbs
- 1/4 mug weed oil
- 6-8 cloves garlic, minced
- Two mugs poultry broth
- 1 1/2 mugs whipping cream
- 1 tsp salt
- 1/2 teaspoon pepper
- 2-3 cups finely shredded Fontina cheese
- One cup chopped fresh basil

Directions:

Boil pasta per package directions. The drainpipe (do not rinse) as well as return right into a pot. Add regarding a tbsp of olive oil and afterwards cover to keep warm. While the pasta is boiling slice poultry and area in zipping leading storage bag, add breadcrumbs tremble as well as use your hands to push crumbs into hen until coated and the majority of the bits are no more loosened. Heat weed oil over medium warmth in a large frying pan. Include poultry as well as toss periodically to make sure that all sides obtain browned. Regarding seven minutes in include garlic and also throw. Attempt to throw this rather than mixing it; this will aid the breadcrumbs remain connected to the poultry. Cook for concerning three, even more, mins (check most significant piece to make sure it is done) as well as remove chicken from pan. Paraventure there is a great deal of oil left in the pan put a ton of it out, otherwise, include poultry juices, cream, pepper and also salt. Give a boil after that adding cheese, remind a boil and gourmet specialist, sometimes blending for five minutes. Include basil and also boil, whisking periodically, for an additional five minutes. Pour over pasta as well as mix up until integrated. Garnish with basil.

Components:

- Two pounds shelled uncooked shrimp.
- Ten Roma tomatoes.
- 3 TBLS of fresh basil.
- Six cloves of garlic.
- 1 1/4 cup of weed oil.
- 2 TBLS of lemon juice.
- 2 TBLS of fresh parsley.
- 2 TBLS of Gewurztraminer.
- 1 TBLS of fresh oregano.
- One teaspoon of salt.
- 1 tsp of pepper.
- Angel hair pasta.

Directions:

- For shrimp and also marinade: Finely slice three cloves of garlic, 2 TBLS of fresh parsley and 1 TBLS of fresh oregano as well as a location in a bowl.
- Include 3/4 mug of olive oil, lemon juice, salt, pepper, white wine.

- Mix.
- Add in shrimp.
- Allow marinating for three hrs.
- Grill on reduced tool warmth.
- Sauce: chop Roma tomatoes, three cloves garlic as well as basil.
- Place sliced tomatoes, garlic and also basil in a sauce frying pan.
- Include 1/2 cup of weed oil.
- Add salt pepper.
- Cook for 5 minutes while stirring.

Integrate: location sauce on prepared angel hair and afterwards include grilled shrimp.

Cannabis Tea

Components:

- 1/2 gram (or more) of your favourite indica, Sativa or any combination of both marijuana.
- 3 Cups of Water
- 2 Tablespoons of butter

Instructions:

First, you will require to navigate 1/2 gram of your favored cannabis as well as grind it up as high as you can.

(Some that I prescribe are Barneys Farm G13 Haze, Green House Seeds Cheese, or LA Confidential). Obtain a small pot and also put 3 cups of water in. Turn the range onto the highest setting possible and bring the water to a boil. Add the 2 tbsps of butter. Add the 1/2 gram of ground-up cannabis. While leaving the range on the most magnificent warmth setup and also having the water violently boiling, mix every few minutes ensuring that any of the marijuana on the side of the put is pushed back right into the water. Note: The factor of making Cannabis tea is to extract the THC from the plant. Because THC is not soluble in water alone, it requires a fatty substance to stick onto under high heat. With the combination of the high temperature from the boiling water after that, the butter that was contributed to the mix the THC can be removed from the marijuana for drinking purposes. All for the cannabis, water as well as butter to boil over warmth for a minimum of thirty minutess. The longer you are willing to wait for the even more THC that will undoubtedly be drawn out. From my experience, thirty-fourty minutes is generally a perfect time. Note: While the water is boiling over warmth, the water will start to evaporate rather quickly. When you return, do NOT turn it on and also stroll away for a fifty per cent the sea or an hr might be gone. Enjoy as well as mix every few minutes and as added water as required to keep that the water level coincides as when you began. After at least thirty minutess, you can run the water with a filter into a cup big enough to hold all the fluid. Now that the THC is eliminated from the marijuana and currently holding on to the butter, you no longer need the green. The marijuana tea will undoubtedly be hot, so be VERY careful and also allow it cool for 5 minutes. Include one of your favoured tea bags to include added taste or beverage as is. Similar to many things consumed by mouth, it will undoubtedly take fiurty-five and sixty minutes for the tea to receive its full result. Note: Be ready to get incredibly stoned. Indeed, even with just a 1/2 gram, this formula is much stronger then it appears. Many individuals have felt the effects for approximately twelve hours from eating the tea. After you have actually made and also fed the marijuana tea, leave a remark listed below informing us how the procedure chose you and how the results were.

Ingredients:

- 10 oz. Cannabis vodka (green dragon).
- 6 oz. Jello mix.
- 16 oz. Steaming water.
- 6 oz. Coldwater.

Directions:

Bring the larger quantity of water to a rolling boil, ultimately adding the Jello mix to the boiling water. Switch off the heat once the Jello has liquified. Next, include the 6 oz. Coldwater (to chill it off for the subsequent stage) and then add the ten. oz of MJ vodka after the virus water. Fill shot glasses or small plastic cups as well as cool for three-five hours, depending on the temperature of the refrigerator.

- 1 cup flour.
- 1/2 mug whole wheat flour.
- 1/4 tsp cinnamon.
- 1/2 tsp baking soft drink.
- 1/2 tsp nutmeg.
- 1/2 tsp salt.
- One egg.
- 1 cup granulated sugar.
- 2/3 mug cannabis-infused olive oil.
- 1/2 mug pecans, sliced.
- 1 1/2 gran smith apples, peeled and grated.
- One gala apple, thinly sliced.

* 15 pecan fifty per cent.
* For the polish:
* 1/4 cup brown sugar.
* 2 tsp marijuana instilled olive oil.
* 2 tsp water.

Instructions:

Heat your stove to 325 degrees Fahrenheit. Lightly layer a 9-inch springtime form pan with nonstick cooking spray. In a medium dish, combine the cinnamon, powders, cooking soft drink, nutmeg and salt until mixed. In a big bowl, blend the egg and also sugar with the 2/3 cup cannabis-infused olive oil. Mix the flour mix right into the egg mixture, as well as include the cut pecans and grated apples. Scratch right into the prepared pan as well as squash the top with a spatula. Prepare the apple slices on top of the edge of the cake, as well as arrange the pecan fifty per cent in one layer in the centre. Make the polish in a little microwavable bowl. Mix the brownish sugar as well as the 2 tsp olive oil as well as water, and microwave in thirty-second periods until the brown sugar is melted. Brush the apples and pecans with fifty per cent of the save the remainder and polish. Bake in the centre of the stove till a toothpick put into the middle of the cake appears tidy, concerning 45 mins. Eliminate from the oven and clean the top of the cosy cake with the remainder of the polish. Get rid of the ring by running a knife around the outside of the cake. Delicately remove the cake from base. Serve with an inside story of vanilla gelato.

Marijuana Cupcakes

Ingredients:

- 1 1/4 cups flour.
- 1/2 -3/ 4 cup sugar (depending upon sweetness desired).
- 1 3/4 tsp cooking powder.
- 1/4 tsp salt.
- 1/3 cup weed butter.
- One egg, beaten.
- 3/4 cup milk.
- 1/2 tsp vanilla.
- 2/3 cup blueberries (or whatever you desire to utilise).
- 1/3 cup chopped unblanched almonds, toasted.

Instructions:

Look completely dry active ingredients together to blend well. Cut the butter in half until the mixture resembles rough crumbs. Blend the egg intensely to bring in the air and also light the eggs. Mix in egg, milk and vanilla and incorporate thoroughly. Include in dry mixture and stir together (some swellings need to remain) and also add the blueberries. Load well-greased muffin tins with batter till two thirds complete. Bake in a preheated 350 ° F broiler for twenty minutes or until done. Note: Makes eighteen large muffins.

Cannabis Brownies

What you need

1. Oil (any oil other than olive oil).

2. 2.5 grams of any Indica or Sativa cannabis (some of which I suggest are Barneys Farm G13 Haze, Green House Seeds Cheese, or LA Confidential).

3. A Grinder.

4. A Filter (coffee filter, pasta strainer).

5. Brownie mix.

6. A Frying pot

7. A timber spoon.

For a whole set of brownies (1 box), a fifty per cent ounce of grace or an ounce of mids is what you need. Grind the marijuana in your grinder or coffee shop several times until it develops into a powder. As soon as the marijuana becomes a powder spread it right onto a frying pan. When drawing out the THC, its a good idea to match the frying pan to the heater dimension for an even cook which is essential. Pour oil straight onto the marijuana powder on the frying pan according to how much the brownie dish asks for. Turn the burner on low (numbers 2-3) up until it starts to simmer and afterwards reduced the stove to the lowest setup (labelled as reduced or simmer). Leave the heater on for two-six hours depending on how much time you have (two hours is average) and stir the marijuana in the oil every thirty minutes with a wooden spoon. At the point when the pot is done, empty the oil blend right into a channel (a coffee channel works fine) to stress all the excess cannabis out. You should be entrusted with a musky brown shading oil with no lawn, stems, or seeds in it. This stuff needs to be expelled because there's no THC left since it was extracted from the oil. Use this oil to make brownies by sticking to the directions on the brownie box. In case you want to make weed brownies using spread instead of oil, keep reading.

What You Need

1. Butter.

2. 2.5 grams of indica or Sativa marijuana (Some that I suggest are Barneys Farm G13 Haze, Green House Seeds Cheese, or LA Confidential).

3. A Grinder.

4. A Filter (coffee filter, pasta filter).

5. Brownie mix.

6. A little pot as well as a bigger pot.

7. A timber spoon.

To make use of butter to remove the THC as well as bake brownies, two pots are called for, one bigger as well as one smaller. The larger one ought to be filled out with clean water and the same dimension as the burner for an even shed. Location the smaller pot inside the larger one as well as throw in 2-3 sticks of butter. Turn the heater on a reduced setup up until the water in the bigger pots starts to simmer. Use your judgment on a high setting med-- overcome to establish a close to simmering once this takes place. The liquid in the larger pot will heat the THC in the cannabis in the smaller pan without shedding it, which can damage the THC, making the brownies ineffective. As soon as done, put the butter via a filter eliminating any seeds, stems, or leftover marijuana bud which is worthless since the THC is now in the butter. Spread this butter throughout the base of a large frying pan as well as pour the brownie mixture on top.

Since you recognise just how to make cannabis brownies making use of the butter technique, tell us how you liked this technique in a remark below.

Cannabis Apple Pecan Galaxy Cake

Ingredients:

- 1/2 mug cannabutter.
- One mug buttermilk.
- Two eggs.
- 2 cups flour.
- One fl. oz. Red food colouring.
- 1.5 tsp. Baking soda.
- 1 tsp. Vanilla remove.
- 1 tbsp. White vinegar.
- 1/3 cup chocolate powder.
- 1 tsp. Common salt.

Instructions:

In a blending bowl mix the softened butter as well as sugar. In a separate bowl, combine the flour, sugar as well as salt and begin to mix into the batter. After it is extensively combined, placed batter in the greased cups as well as bake for twenty/twenty-five minutes.

Cannabis Chocolate Pudding

ingredients:

- Two mugs marijuana milk.
- One box split-second dessert mix, chocolate (14 oz).
- 1/2 tsp ground cinnamon.
- 1/2 cup frozen whipped topping, defrosted.

Directions:

Beat the pudding mix, marijuana milk and cinnamon with a whisk for concerning two minutes. Mix in the thawed out whipped covering until entirely mixed. Refrigerate for regarding thirty minutes, and delight in!

Cannabis Cashew Cookies

Ingredients:

Crust:

- 4 tbsp (1/2 stick) cannabutter
- One mug flour (can make use of cannabis flour as well, yet may influence consistency).
- 1/3 mug packed brown sugar.
- 1/4 tsp. salt.

Covering:

- 1/2 mug butterscotch chips.
- 1/4 cup light corn syrup.
- Two tablespoons. Cannabutter.
- One cup salted cashews.

Direction.

Preheat the broiler to 350 degrees Fahrenheit as well as placed sugar in a medium blending bowl. Assimilate two tablespoons. Cannabutter till the uniformity resembles crumbs. Next include the flour and salt, mixing thoroughly. Press into an ungreased frying pan and bake for elevn-twelve minutes. In a different container, thaw the butterscotch, corn syrup as well as 2 tbsp. Do not boil it, simmer. Pour over the crust, subsequently adding the cashews and let high. Appreciate.

ingredients:

- One cup softened marijuana butter.
- 2.75 mugs flour.
- 1.5 mugs sugar.
- One egg.
- 1 tsp. vanilla.
- 1 tsp. baking soda.

Directions:

Preheat the oven to 375 degrees Fahrenheit. Next, in a blending bowl mix the flour, cooking powder and also baking soft drink. In a separate yet more significant dish, mix the softened butter and sugar up until the consistency is smooth, consequently mixing in the egg and vanilla extract. After this is done, slowly mix in the flour, baking soft drink and also baking powder, rolling the dough into little rounds as well as a place on an unbuttered flat pan, cooking for eight to ten minutes.

ingredients:

- 1 cup flour
- 1/2 mug entire wheat flour
- 1/4 tsp cinnamon
- 1/2 tsp cooking soft drink
- 1/2 tsp nutmeg
- 1/2 tsp salt
- One egg
- 1 cup granulated sugar
- 2/3 mug cannabis-infused olive oil
- 1/2 mug pecans, sliced
- 1 1/2 gran smith apples, peeled off and also grated
- One gala apple, thinly sliced
- 15 pecan fifty per cents
- For the polish:
- 1/4 cup brown sugar
- 2 tsp marijuana-infused olive oil
- 2 tsp water

Instructions:

In a tool dish, combine the cinnamon, powders, baking soda, nutmeg as well as salt up until blended. This stuff needs to be expelled as there is no THC left since it was extracted from the oil. Make the polish in a little microwavable dish. Mix the brown sugar and the 2 tsp olive oil and water, as well as a microwave in thirty 2nd periods till the brownish sugar is melted. Brush the apples and also pecans with half of the save the rest and even glaze. Bake in the facility of the oven till a toothpick put right into the centre of the cake comes out clean, about fourty-five minutes. Eliminate from the oven and brush the top of the warm cake with the rest of the glaze.

Ingredients:

- 3/4 cup cannabis-infused olive oil.
- 1/3 cup honey.
- 1 3/4 cup ripe bananas, mashed up.
- 3/4 tsp salt.
- Four cups uncooked routine oats.
- 1/2 cup nuts, sliced.
- 1/2 mug raisins (Optional: change with chocolate chips).

Directions.

In a tool dish mix with each other, the honey and also oil until well blended. Mix in the mashed bananas and salt, mix well. Permit to cool down for 5 minutes as well as move from baking sheet to cooling down shelf.

Ingredients:

- Six tablespoons. (3/4 stick) cannabutter.
- 1.5 cups flour.
- One cup of cane sugar.
- Two large eggs.
- 1/2 cup milk (canna milk works too).
- 1/2 mug cane sugar (again).
- 1/2 cup sliced walnuts (optional).
- One juiced lemon.

- 1 tsp. Lemon enthusiasm (carefully grated lemon peel).
- 1 tsp. Cooking powder.
- 1/2 tsp. salt (or lemon salt).

Instructions:

In a tiny bowl, blend the flour, salt (or lemon salt) and also cooking powder, till combined thoroughly. In a separate yet larger bowl, mix the softened cannabutter, eggs as well as mug of sugar with each other. At the end of the baking time in the oven, mix the continuing to be 1/2 cup walking stick sugar as well as the juice of the lemon.

Orange Cake

Ingredients:

- 2/3 mug marijuana-infused olive oil.
- Three blood oranges (seasonal, but regular oranges will function ok.).
- One cup of cane sugar.
- Three eggs.
- 1/2 mug buttermilk or unflavored yoghurt.
- 1 3/4 mug routine flour.
- 1 1/2 tsp. Cooking powder.
- 1/4 tsp baking soft drink.
- 1/4 tsp. salt.
- Whipped cream to for offering, if wanted.

Directions:

With the remaining orange, reduced it in half as well as juice it into a determining cup. Include the buttermilk or yoghurt to this blend until it is 2/3 of a mug integrated.

Now, while mixing in the eggs as well as olive oil into the dish of sugar and also orange rhine, additionally add the buttermilk/orange juice blend as well as blend this all together.

Chocolate Milkshake

Components:

- Three scoops chocolate ice cream (medicated for extra potency).
- 1/2 mug canna milk.
- Chocolate syrup to preference.

Instructions:

Put all active ingredients in a blender as well as mix up until smooth and also thoroughly blended consistency. For extra delicious chocolate flavour and presentation, line the inside of a glass with delicious chocolate syrup, pour the milkshake in as well as enjoy a yummy, medical treatment.

Banana Blueberry Healthy Smoothie

Ingredients:

- 5 oz. Canna milk.
- Three scoops vanilla gelato.
- 2 oz. Espresso or robust coffee.
- 1 tbsp. Cream cheese.
- You have powdered delicious chocolate.
- Whipped lotion (medicated whipped cream works too.

Instructions:

Initially, put the 2 ounces of coffee in a blender or food processor, consequently pouring in the 5 ounces of canna milk. Now include the lotion cheese, in addition to the gelato and also mix up until the consistency is smooth. After it is combined, fill a high glass about 1/3 full, after that layer with some whipped cream, a cleaning of chocolate, complied with by even more of the blended mix, even more, whipped cream and the last cleaning of delicious chocolate. Enjoy as well as remember that this is going to medicate you entirely, as a result of the amount of canna milk, so plan on relaxing and sleeping. A great reward after dinner.

Cinnamon Coffee Cake

ingredients:

Cake:

- 1 1/4 mugs flour (cannabis flour for extra effectiveness).
- 1/4 mug cannabutter.
- 1/2 cup sugar.
- 1/4 cup sour cream.
- 1/3 cup canna milk (or regular milk).
- Two eggs beat a little.
- 2 tsp cooking powder.
- 1.5 tsp. Cinnamon.
- Topping:
- 1/3 mug flour.
- 1/3 mug brown sugar.
- 1/4 mug cannabutter.
- 1 tsp. Cinnamon.

Instructions:

After thoroughly blending, pour the batter onto an eight or 9-inch greased/buttered baking frying pan. After this combine the flour and also brown sugar for the covering in a dish, blending in the cannabutter and likewise cinnamon after.

Canna Flat Bread

Ingredients:

The Dough:

- Two mugs marijuana flour (see a dish on-site).
- Two tablespoons. Granulated sugar.
- 4 tsp. Baking powder.
- 1 tsp. Salt.
- 3 tbsp. Cannabutter.
- 3/4 mug milk (medicated for added effectiveness.
- The Filling up:
- 4 tbsp. Cannabutter.
- One cup of brown sugar.
- 3 tsp. Cinnamon.
- The Luster:
- 1/2 mug powdered sugar.
- 1/4 mug milk (medicated for extra effectiveness.

Directions:

First of all, preheat your stove to 375 degrees. In a tiny to medium-sized blending bowl, combine all the filling ingredients up until it forms a crumbly, but well-mixed blend (tip: it aids to soften the cannabutter initially). Next, spread fifty per cent of this blend over all-time low of a

9"x 9" frying pan, or closest dimension you have. Currently, in a big blending dish, incorporate the cannabis flour, sugar, cooking powder and also salt as well as mix together thoroughly. Slowly begin to include much progressively softened cannabutter a little each time up until all-around combined and also ultimately blend in the milk. Spread some of the canna flour on a cutting board or comparable surface as well as an overlay into a 1/4" thick rectangular shape. Spread it on top of the moving rectangle of the batter with the other half of your filling. Next off, overlay the rectangular shape up right into a log and cut into eighteen equivalent sectors or twelve if you choose bigger rolls. Bake for twenty-five/thirty minutes on 375 levels Fahrenheit. While this is cooking, incorporate the canna milk (or regular milk) and powdered sugar in a dish and also. Spread out on top of the rolls when out of the oven. Allow cool a min or two and prepare to get genuinely medicated.

Tiramisu Milk Shake

ingredients:

- One mug canna milk.
- 2 cups fresh blueberries.
- One cut banana.
- One cup of strawberry yoghurt.

Directions:

Place all components in a blender or food processor and also blend up until the consistency is smooth. Pour, take pleasure in and also offer.

Ingredients:

- Four mugs cannabis flour (see a dish on-site).
- 1.5 cups canna milk (see recipe on-site).
- 1.5 tablespoon. Granulated sugar.
- 1/2 tbsp. cooking powder.
- 1/2 tbsp. Baking soda.
- 2 tsp. Vinegar (white or cider tastes ideal).

Instructions:

Combine the canna flour, sugar, cooking powder and also baking soda, mixing extensively. Next, combine the vinegar and also canna milk, blending, before including to the dry components. For a powerful reward, use as salute with cannabutter on top.

Canna Extra Pound Cake

These marijuana sugar squares with sea salt as well as a wonderfully decadent reward for you to try. The most effective part is that they're straightforward to make.

ingredients:

- One mug cannabutter (2 sticks or 1/2 pound).
- One mug light whipping cream.
- 1 1/2 mugs brown sugar.
- 3/4 cup sugar.
- 1/2 mug light corn syrup.
- 1/4 mug dark corn syrup.
- 1 tsp. Sea salt.
- 1 tsp. Vanilla.

Instructions:

Venture out a big pan (a minimum of 1/2 or 3/4 gallon ability) and also butter all-time low and sides. If you have extra, you can utilise cannabutter to do this. Currently, add the 1/2 pound of cannabutter as well as melt it on deficient heat. You do not want to use a tool or a high temperature, because you will shed butter and therefore waste precious cannabinoids. As soon as the butter is belted, add the brown sugar, sugar, both corn syrups and the light whipping cream, adding each ingredient a little at once and also mixing in a while doing so. Since all your parts are in, you can quickly increase the warm to medium-high, yet no more, and also bring the mix to a boil, stirring off and on while doing so. When it first starts to steam, decrease the warm to a tool or listed below medium and remain to cook, stirring periodically until the mix gets to 248 degrees Fahrenheit. As soon as the combination has reached 248 degrees, eliminate it from the warmth as well as stir in the tsp. After this is complete, but the mixture right into a 9" cooking pan that has been lined with aluminium foil and the foil has been greased with butter. Make sure it cools entirely before you make use of to aluminium foil to raise the block of caramel out of the frying pan.

Ingredients:

- 1 1/2 tablespoon. EXTREMELY POTENT marijuana-infused butter.
- 2 1/2 cups self-raising flour.
- One pinch of salt.
- 1 tsp. Cooking soda.

- 3 1/4 tablespoon margarine.
- 1 1/2 tbsp castor sugar.
- 2/3 cup milk.
- One mug dried fruit of your option.

Directions:

Currently, blend the flour, salt, cooking soda and margarine into a big mixing bowl. Now, include the milk/butter mixture as well as sugar right into the blending bowl that has the various other active ingredients as well as steadily massaged it together. Spread the dough onto a level surface evenly, until it regards 1" thick. It must be saltless if you want the best taste. Directly, I like to make it extra-potent, yet for this recipe, and butter from a dispensary should be high because you'll be utilising all of it.

Ingredients:

- One extra pound cannabutter (4 sticks).
- 3.5 cups all-round flour.
- One mug powdered sugar.
- One tablespoon. Vanilla extract.

Instructions:

Either let the margarine sit out until softened or microwave on the shallow setting, till totally softened, however not liquid. After that, in a large blending bowl, include the spread, vanilla and also powdered sugar and blend extensively with each other. After you have done this, blend in the flour at regarding one mug each time, blending it in after everyone. Putting all the powder in simultaneously will certainly create clumps and issues when attempting to get it to a smooth consistency.

After all the dough is extensively mixed, create the cookies into desired forms on the cookie sheet, ensuring to keep them around an inch high, so they don't get as well hard as well as crispy. Preheat the stove to 375 as well as when it's all set, placed the cookies in the oven for ten to twelve minutes, or until gold brownish ahead. While still cosy, sprinkle more powdered sugar on top. Let trendy as well as take pleasure in one of the most potent cookies you've ever had.

Delicious Chocolate Space Cake

Marijuana-infused banana bread is liked by Cannabis individuals around. It is an excellent means to medicate as well as is not extremely rich as well as beautiful as several edibles can be. The best method to make banana bread is to make use of medicated butter or margarine. Nonetheless, it can also be made using very carefully ground Cannabis.

Products

- You are cooking grease.
- One glass loaf-baking frying pan.
- One stirring spoon.

Active ingredients.

- Two mugs flour.
- Three bananas.

- 1/2 mug sour cream or hefty light whipping cream.
- One cup of walking stick sugar.
- Two medium-sized eggs.
- 1 tsp baking soft drink.
- 1/2 cup chopped walnuts.
- 1/2 tsp vanilla extract.
- 1/2 cup CannaButter (potency of the bread relies on the effectiveness of the butter).

Directions

Beat the softened butter, eggs, sugar and also sour cream (or whipping lotion) in a big mixing dish. Next, slowly yet progressively, add in the flour, mixing it in after each addition to the meal. When you have actually blended in all the flour, add the walnuts.

Marijuana Cheesecake

Cannabis-infused cheesecake is one of the tastiest pleasant edibles available. The best method to make medicated cheesecake is to utilise hash oil or honey oil as well as thaw it gradually right into the butter that is asked for in the dish. Nevertheless, it can additionally be used the standard CannaButter recipe

Ingredients:

- 1 3/4 cups carefully crushed graham crackers.
- 1/4 mug carefully cut walnuts or pecans.
- 1/2 tsp cinnamon.
- 1/2 cup melted butter.
- 4 - 6 grams of hash oil or honey oil (BHO).
- Loading.

- 3 8 oz bags of softened cream cheese.
- One cup fine granulated sugar.
- 2 tbsp flour.
- 1 tsp vanilla extract.
- 1/2 tsp finely shredded lemon peel.
- Two medium-sized eggs.
- One egg yolk.
- 1/4 cup milk.

Instructions

Crust

Gradually melt honey oil or hash oil right into the 1/2 cup of butter only as you would certainly when making normal CannaButter. Currently, mix in the BHO butter.

We are filling up

Whip the cream cheese, flour, sugar, vanilla as well as the lemon peel in a mixing dish with an electric mixer. Include in the two eggs as well as the egg yolk with each other as well as wait while it is progressively mixed in. Now, gradually mix in the milk.

Marijuana Truffles

One of the much more usual marijuana edibles discovered at dispensaries, truffles is an incredibly yummy way to medicate for many people. Nevertheless, these decadent infants are not unique to dispensaries. You can make your very own right in your kitchen area.

Ingredients:

- 12 oz. semi-sweet delicious chocolate morsels.
- 1/4 mug very great granulated sugar.
- Two ruined egg yolks.
- One mug finely sliced walnuts, almonds or hazelnuts.
- 1/3 cup liqueur (Kahlua).
- 4 tbsp CannaButter.

Directions:

When the butter has melted in, stirring constantly, include in the sugar until it liquefies in the chocolate and also butter. When you do this, add the egg yolks with the chocolate right into the pot, blending it in thoroughly. Mix in the almonds and liqueur as well as put onto a glass brownie frying pan.

Chocolate Chip Cookies

Cannabis cookies are remarkably good to eat, can be one of the new potent edibles available, are valued relatively (typically in between $5 and also $20 at the majority of dispensaries, depending on dose) as well as have long-lasting results. Pot brownies are generally not prescribed for daytime usage although, depending on the dosage, it is feasible to operate while medicated.

Dish:

- Chocolate chips (one 12 ounce bag).
- Brownish Sugar (1/2 mug).
- Egg (1 tool size).
- Granulated sugar (1/4 cup).

- Baking soda (1/2 tsp).
- Flour (1 1/3 cup).
- Salt (1/2 tsp).
- Cannabis butter (1/2 mug).

Note: The dosage depends on the effectiveness of your marijuana spread. Preheat your stove to 375 F. Next, blend both of the sugars, margarine and also egg in a large bowl. Do this by hand. Next off, hereafter is stirred up, include the sodium bicarbonate as well as salt. After that, slowly include the flour a bit at a time, blending it in after each enhancement. Now, add in the chocolate chips, mixing continuously. As soon as this combination is thoroughly combined, you will undoubtedly require to oil a cookie sheet. Use your clean hands to move around 1-inch rounds of treat batter as well as a place on the treated sheet approximately 2 inches aside from each other. Place the treated sheet in the broiler and cook for ten to twelve minutes, allow tremendously and appreciate your medication.

Cannabis Pumpkin Muffins

Ingredients:

- 1/2 mug canned pumpkin puree
- 1 egg
- 3/4 mug milk
- 2 Tbsp. canola oil
- 2 mugs cake flour
- 3 tsp. baking powder
- 1 tsp. ground ginger
- 1 +1/ 2 tsp. cinnamon
- 1/2 tsp. ground cloves
- 1/4 tsp. salt

- 1/2 mug dark brownish sugar, loaded
- 1 cup fresh cranberries, finely cut
- 1/4 cup granulated sugar
- Weed Butter

Instructions:

Sift with each other flour, baking powder, ginger, cloves, as well as salt in a large blending dish. Spoon into twelve muffin cups. Allow sitting in a frying pan 1 minute, after that roll in granulated sugar while still cosy.

Marijuana Orange Dark Chocolate Chip Cookies

Ingredients:

- 1/2 c weed butter
- 1/2 c butter flavour shortening
- 3/4 c white sugar
- 3/4 c light brown sugar
- Two eggs
- 2 tsp Mexican vanilla
- grated rind from one orange
- juice from one orange
- 2 1/4 c all function flour
- 1 tsp cooking soda
- 1 tsp salt
- Two mugs Hershey's Special Dark delicious chocolate chips

Directions

Preheat stove to 350. Silpat cookie sheets, use parchment, or oil lightly. Cream the weed butter, reducing, brownish sugar, white sugar, orange juice, as well as vanilla up until light and also fluffy. Add eggs one at a time defeating well after each addition. Combine the dry components as well as the orange peel and stir into the creamed mixture. Fold in delicious chocolate chips lightly as well as fresh for twenty minutes approximately.

Visit rounded teaspoonfuls on a cooking sheet and cook eight-ten minutes till light golden brown and also still soft, yet embedded in the middle. Allow cool on the treated sheet for five minutes and after that dispose of to cooling down shelf or counter 3-4 dozen cookies.

Marijuana Cranberry and also Macadamia Nut Cookies

Ingredients:

- 2 1/4 cups all-purpose flour.
- 1 tsp baking soda.
- 1/2 tsp baking powder.
- 1/2 tsp salt.
- 3/4 cup weed butter, room temperature.
- 1 cup of sugar.
- 1/2 cup milk.
- 1 tsp vanilla remove.
- 1 1/2 mugs approximately cut Maltesers/whoppers/malted milk rounds.

Instructions:

Preheat the stove to 350F and line a cooking sheet with parchment paper. In a tool dish, blend flour, cooking powder, cooking soft drink and salt. In a huge dish, cream with each other weed butter and sugar up until light and fluffy. Stir in milk and vanilla, after that slowly blend in the flour mix. Do not overmix; stir just until no streaks of flour continue to be. Combination in the cut Maltesers/Whoppers/Malted Milk Balls. Go down right into 1-inch spheres (tbsp sized balls) on the prepared flat pan as well as bake for twelve-forteen minutes, up until lightly browned. High on baking sheet for two-three minutes, then transfer to a cake rack to cool totally.

ingredients:

- Two mugs all-round flour.
- 1 1/2 teaspoons cooking powder.
- 1/4 teaspoon baking soda.
- 1 1/2 tsp ground cinnamon.
- 1/2 cup weed butter, softened.
- 1 cup white sugar.
- 3 tbsps real syrup.
- One egg.
- 1/2 mug white sugar.
- 1/4 cup maple sugar.

Instructions:

Preheat stove to 350 levels F (175 degrees C). Stir together the flour, cooking powder, baking soft drink, and cinnamon. Reserve. In a considerable bowl, cream with each other the margarine as well as 1 cup of white sugar up until light and cosy. In a small dish, mix the continuing to be 1/2 mug white sugar and the maple sugar. Roll dough right into 1-inch spheres, as well as roll the areas in the sugar blend.

Bake eight-ten minutes in the preheated stove. Cookies will certainly be crackly on the top and also look wet between. Dispose of from treat sheets to chill off on cake rack.

Marijuana Caramel Walnut Dream Bars

ingredients:

- One box yellow cake mix.
- Three tablespoons weed butter softened.
- One egg.
- Fourteen ounces of sweetened compressed milk.
- One egg.
- 1 tsp pure vanilla extract.
- 1/2 mug walnuts carefully ground.
- 1/2 mug finely ground toffee bits.

Directions:

Incorporate cake mix, weed butter and one egg in a mixing bowl then blend up until crumbly. In another mixing dish incorporate milk, continuing to be an egg, remove, walnuts and also toffee bits. Bake for thirty-five minutes.

Iced Marshmallow Cookies

ingredients:

- 1/2 mug weed butter.
- 2 (1-ounce) squares unsweetened delicious chocolate.
- One huge egg.
- One mug loaded brownish sugar.
- One teaspoon vanilla extract.
- 1/2 tsp cooking soda.

* 1 1/2 mugs all-round flour.
* 1/2 mug milk.
* 1 (16-ounce) package of enormous marshmallows.
* Delicious chocolate Icing:
* 6 tbsps bitter baking cacao.
* 3 tbsps weed butter, melted.
* 2 cups powdered sugar.
* 4 to 6 tbsp warm water.

Directions:

Preheat stove to 350 ° F(175 ° C). Lightly grease treat sheets or line with parchment paper. Thaw weed spread and delicious chocolate in a little powerful pan over low warmth; blend to blend. Dispose of from heat; cool. Beat egg, brown sugar, vanilla and also cooking soft drink in the big bowl up until light as well as fluffy. Blend in the chocolate blend and even flour until smooth. Slowly beat in milk to make fire, cake batter-like dough. Drop dough by spoonfuls 2-inches apart onto ready cookie sheets. Cook ten to twelve minutes or until firm in a facility. Area halved marshmallow, reduced side down, onto each baked cookie. Return to oven one min or just up until marshmallow is warm sufficient to stick to the cookie. For Chocolate Icing: Combine all components in bowl as well as beat by hand till smooth.

Marijuana Brown-eyes

ingredients:

* 1 c. Weed butter.
* Three tablespoons. Sugar.
* 1 tsp. Almond essence.

- 2 c. Flour.
- 1/2 tsp. salt.
- Frosting:
- 1 c. Powdered sugar.
- 2 tbsp. Cocoa.
- Almond halves.
- 2 tbsp. Warm water.
- 1/2 tsp. vanilla.

Instructions:

Include sugar, extract, flour as well as salt. Location on the cookie sheet and flatten a little with a thumbprint.

Frosting:

Combine sugar as well as cacao. Add the water and vanilla. Put 1/2 tsp of icing on each cookie with almond in the centre.

Marijuana Peanut Butter Cup Cookies

Ingredients:

- 1 3/4 mugs versatile flour
- 1/2 tsp salt
- 1 tsp baking soft drink
- 1/2 cup weed butter, softened
- 1/2 mug white sugar
- 1/2 mug peanut butter
- 1/2 mug loaded brown sugar
- One egg, beaten
- One teaspoon vanilla remove

- 2 tbsps milk
- 40 miniature chocolate-covered peanut butter cups, unwrapped

Instructions:

Preheat broiler to 375 degrees F (190 levels C). Sift with each other the flour, salt as well as baking soda; set aside.

Salve with each other the weed spread, sugar, peanut margarine and also brown sugar up until cushioned.

Beat in the egg, vanilla as well as milk. Add the flour combination; mix well. Forming into 40 spheres and also location each right into an ungreased mini muffin frying pan Bake at 375 degrees for concerning eight minutes. Remove from the oven and quickly push a tiny peanut butter cup right into each ball. Excellent and also meticulously get rid of the pan.

Marijuana Butterscotch Space Pops

ingredients:

- One mug sugar 1/3 cup corn syrup 1/2 cup water
- 1/4 tsp cream of tartar 1/4 to 1 teaspoon flavour
- fluid food coloring 1 to 2 teaspoon(s) citric acid (optional).

Directions:

Prepare either a marble slab or an upside-down cookie sheet (air underneath the layer will undoubtedly assist the candy is cooling faster), by covering it with parchment paper and also spraying it with oil. In your pan, over medium warm, mix the sugar, corn syrup, water, and lotion of tartar with a wood spoon till the sugar crystals liquify. Continue to mix, making use of a bread brush wetted with cosy water to dissolve any sugar crystals holding on to the sides of the frying pan, then stop stirring as quickly as the syrup begins to steam. Place the candy thermostat in the pan, being careful not to let it touch all-time low or sides, and also allow the syrup boil without mixing up until the thermostat reaches 300degrees F (hard-crack stage). Get rid of the pan from the warm promptly and allow the syrup cool to concerning 275degrees F before including taste, shade, marijuana tincture and citric acid (adding it sooner triggers the majority of the feeling to prepare away).

Care be mindful. The sugar syrup is incredibly warm. If you melt yourself, run cold water over your hand for several minutes, but do not use ice. Functioning swiftly, put the syrup right into the ready moulds as well as let cool down for around ten minutes. If you're not using molds, pour little (2-inch) circles onto the prepared marble slab or cookie sheet and location a lollipop stick in each one, turning the rod to be sure it's covered with sweet. Let the lollipops cool down for at least ten minutes, till they are tight. Shop in a cool, dry place. You can just put tiny circles of syrup onto a greased cookie sheet and also location sticks in the middle to make stands out. Cooking sweet syrup to the preferred temperature indicates attaining a specific ratio of sugar to wetness in the fresh. On a humid day, as soon as the candy has cooled to the point where it is no much longer evaporating moisture right into the air, it can start reabsorbing wetness from the air.

Frequently Asked Question: *Why do I add corn syrup?* Corn syrup acts as an interfering representative in this as well as several various other candy dishes.

What is the cream of tartar? Lotion of tartar, or potassium bitartrate, is a fine white powder that is a byproduct of the wine-making process. It is stemmed from argol, or tartar, which forms naturally throughout the fermentation of grape juice into a glass of wine as well as is deposited on the sides of the glass of wine barrels. It serves in this dish because it is an acid, one more kind of interfering representative which inverts sucrose into fructose as well as glucose as well as thereby aids to stop condensation of the sugar syrup.

Why do I add citric acid? Citric acid, sold as colourless crystals or powder, is an optional ingredient that includes flavour to fruit-flavoured candies. The sour covering on the super-sour sweets that are so popular today is a mixture of citric acid as well as sugary substance.

It can be found in many supermarkets, craft shops, and cooking supply stores occasionally it is kept in the Kosher nourishment section and is called sour salt. It is likewise what provides fruits such as lemons as well as limes their sour inclination.

Why do I have to stop mixing after the syrup starts to boil? At this point, you have liquified the crystal structure of the sugar. Mixing or other agitation is among the many factors that can motivate the fructose and also glucose particles in your syrup to rejoin as well as create sucrose crystals of table sugar.

Why do I wash down the sides of the pan? Again, the sugar crystals are liquified now at the same time. A solitary "seed" crystal of sugar holding on to the bottom of the pot might fall in and is an additional factor that can urge recrystallisation. Some pointers for flavouring hard candy You can utilise seasoning essences that are available in the cooking materials area of your neighbourhood.

Supermarket, such as vanilla, almond, anise, maple, as well as lemon. About 1 tsp of this kind of flavour must suffice for a batch of lollipops. There are likewise highly-concentrated flavours especially for candy making, readily available online or in specialised stores.

The taste selections are practically limitless. These typically come in little 1-dram (1 teaspoon) containers, and also 1/4 teaspoon should be sufficient to flavour a batch of lollipops. It's an excellent idea to have the tastes and even colours that you will contribute to your candy distributed and ready beforehand. You will certainly need to function quickly as soon as the syrup gets to the hard-crack stage since it will solidify rapidly!

When utilising more powerful tastes such as cinnamon, mint, and also cherry, you can make use of a percentage (concerning 1/4 teaspoon). Subtler flavours such as lemon, strawberry, peach, and orange call for even more (1/2 to 1 tsp.).

You can include about 1/2 teaspoon of vanilla remove with these flavours to accent them and add a creamy taste. Save the stronger flavours for last, or they might infect the other sets if you are making numerous sets.

Make sure to clean all-determining and blending spoons in between batches too. - Hard-Crack Stage 300degrees F - 310degrees F Sugar concentration:

99% The hard-crack phase is the highest possible temperature you are most likely to see defined in a sweet dish. At these temperature levels, there is virtually no water left in the syrup. Go down a little of the molten sugar in cold water, and it will undoubtedly form hard, brittle threads that break when curved.

CAUTION: To avoid burns, enable the syrup to cool down in the cold water for a couple of moments before touching it!

Do Not Go Yet; One Last Thing To Do

On the off chance that you appreciated this book or thought that it was useful I'd be grateful on the off chance that you'd post a short survey on Amazon. Your support really does make a distinction and I read all the reviews personally so I can get your feedback and make this book far better.

Thanks again for your support!

www.ingramcontent.com/pod-product-compliance
Lightning Source LLC
Chambersburg PA
CBHW070819250726
48662CB00003B/1013